GROWING UP
UNDIAGNOSED

Becca Lory Hector

GROWING UP UNDIAGNOSED

Surviving Childhood in New York City as an Undiagnosed Autistic

The Disability Studies Collection

Collection Editors

**Dr Damian Mellifont
&
Dr Jennifer Smith-Merry**

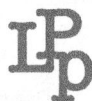

LPp

For you, Mom. Because we simply cannot know what we do not know.

First published in 2024 by Lived Places Publishing

British Library Cataloguing in Publication Data
A CIP record for this book is available from the British Library

ISBN: 9781915271365 (pbk)
ISBN: 9781915271389 (ePDF)
ISBN: 9781915271372 (ePUB)

Cover design by Fiachra McCarthy
Book design by Rachel Trolove of Twin Trail Design
Typeset by Newgen Publishing UK

Lived Places Publishing
Long Island
New York 11789

www.livedplacespublishing.com

Abstract

What does growing up with autism truly feel like, and how can a parent best support their Autistic child? *Growing Up Undiagnosed* is a poignant, insightful guide written by Becca Lory Hector, aimed at providing neurotypical parents with a deeper understanding of the Autistic experience.

This book is a treasure trove for parents, especially for those seeking to comprehend and cater to their child's unique needs. Becca Lory Hector shares her personal journey with autism, offering an intimate glimpse into the sensory sensitivities, social intricacies, and often misunderstood aspects of living in an Autistic body. Through her experiences, she illuminates the challenges and triumphs of growing up Autistic, providing practical advice and compassionate guidance to parents.

Growing Up Undiagnosed is more than a memoir; it is a roadmap for parents who are dedicated to understanding and supporting their Autistic children. It addresses the critical question of how to ensure that an Autistic child not only copes but thrives in a world that's not always accommodating to their needs. The book empowers parents to be the best advocates for their children, ensuring they have every opportunity for a happy, successful life. It's a must-read for any parent who wonders what it's like to grow up with autism and is committed to giving their child the brightest future possible.

Keywords

Autism; sensory sensitivities; neurodiversity; parental guidance; Autistic experiences; social invalidation; emotional support; advocacy; disability; mental health; identity; empowerment; New York City

Acknowledgments

This book is a culmination of not just my efforts, but the support, guidance, and encouragement of many, many people over the years. First and foremost, my deepest gratitude goes to my husband and support person, Antonio Hector, who ensures that our entire household feels loved and cared for. Without you doing the endless list of things that you are good at, I could not do the one thing that I am good at. To my mentor, Angela Lauria from The Author Incubator, without whom this book would not exist at all, I am grateful for your insightful guidance and relentless accountability, which kept me motivated at every stage of this journey. My heartfelt thanks also go to the folks in my life who lived through life's lessons with me and those who shared their wisdom with me along the way. Last, but not least, I am grateful to the countless Autistic authors whose works came before mine and gave me the courage to add my stories to our growing voice.

About the author

Becca Lory Hector is an openly Autistic professional on a mission to close the disability gap in leadership by working with companies to attract and retain disabled talent via their diversity, equity, inclusion, and belonging (DEIB) initiatives. Becca was identified Autistic as an adult and has since become a dedicated autism and neurodiversity advocate, researcher, consultant, speaker, and author. In addition to her work in DEIB, she is focused on Autistic quality of life research and her personal development course called "Self-Defined Living: A Path to a Quality Autistic Life". All with the goal of spreading acceptance, building understanding, and encouraging self-advocacy. She is also an animal lover with a special affinity for cats who spends most of her "free" time with her many animals, her husband Antonio, and her emotional support animal, Sir Walter Underfoot.

Content warning

This book contains explicit references to, and descriptions of, situations that may cause distress.

This includes references to and descriptions of:

- Suicidal thoughts, intentions, and actions;
- Substance use and abuse, illicit drugs, and prescription medication;
- Hospitalization and medical settings; and
- Ableism, discrimination, and micro-aggressions.

Every effort has been made to provide more specific content warnings before relevant chapters, but please be aware that references to potentially distressing topics occur frequently and throughout the book.

Contents

Content warning   ix

Learning objectives   xii

Chapter 1   The answers start here   1

Chapter 2   Cat lover   7

Chapter 3   Twice exceptional   13

Chapter 4   Library kid   23

Chapter 5   Autistic naivety   31

Chapter 6   Setting expectations   43

Chapter 7   Chicken nuggets and fries   51

Chapter 8   Sensory hellscapes   59

Chapter 9   The price of pretending   69

Chapter 10 Brightness and burnout   79

Chapter 11 Discovering regulation   87

Chapter 12 A life you don't need a vacation from   97

Suggested discussion topics   109

References   110

Recommended reading   112

Index   113

Learning objectives

This book is designed to support readers in:

1. Understanding autism from a personal perspective: gain insights into the experiences and challenges faced by Autistic individuals, through the lens of the author's personal journey;

2. Sensory sensitivities and social challenges: learn about the sensory sensitivities and social intricacies that come with being Autistic and understand how they impact daily living and interactions;

3. Support strategies for parents: acquire knowledge on practical strategies and approaches for supporting Autistic children, focusing on emotional support, advocacy, and creating accommodating environments; and

4. Advocacy and empowerment: understand the importance of advocacy for and with Autistic individuals, and how to empower them to lead fulfilling lives while embracing their neurodiversity.

1
The answers start here

I was identified as Autistic at the ripe old age of 36 and my diagnosis saved my life.

It was a gorgeous, sunny, spring afternoon in May when my life changed forever. I remember the weather in particular as it's been an enthusiasm of mine since childhood. As I sat in the passenger seat of my mother's Jeep digesting the news, I noted that it was an especially low-humidity day, sunny but not hot—an anomaly for the time of year in New York.

I looked over at my mother. She, too, was processing the report we had just heard. Tears brimming her eyes, she turned to me and asked, "Are you okay?"

I thought about it. For most of my 36 years, I was NOT okay. In fact, I spent a good chunk of those years angry, sad, confused, resentful, lost, and very much wishing it would all go away. Suicidal ideations became the norm for me somewhere around eight years old. The planning, wishing, and hoping for the courage to do it didn't become the norm until my 20s. For three decades, I had failure after failure, followed by deep depressive episodes, only broken by panic attacks as my anxiety raged. Was I okay?

"No, I'm not. And I haven't been," I answered, "but maybe now I will be?"

That evening, as we sat for dinner in a room filled only with the sound of forks on plates and the TV droning "Law & Order SVU" in the background, my mom voiced her regret. "I wish I had known. I'm sorry I didn't do better."

But how could she have known? Autism wasn't a conversation in the 1980s. As a child, I was just the quirky girl who read too much and struggled with change, sensory inputs, and social cues. My hyperlexia was seen as a gift, my emotional challenges as mere childhood phases. Hyperlexia refers to the condition where children show an intense early interest in letters and are capable of decoding words accurately but without understanding their meaning. The research acknowledges that children with autism and hyperlexia follow a unique pathway towards literacy. Up to 20 per cent of Autistic children demonstrate hyperlexia (Macdonald, Luk, and Quintin, 2022).

If you're reading this, maybe you're a bit like my client Penny from Brooklyn, a mother to an Autistic child who told me she is worried about her child's future and wonders if there is anything she could be doing differently. Maybe, like Penny, you discovered this book a few years after your child's autism diagnosis, seeking understanding, guidance, and perhaps solace in another's journey. Perhaps, like Penny, you've embraced your child's uniqueness but are still navigating the winding path of raising an Autistic child. If that's you, I hope my story offers you the companionship and insights I wish my mom and I could have had back then.

Born in the Bronx, NY in the late 1970s, I was to be my mom's first and only child. She and my dad were high school sweethearts who were starting a family like you are "supposed to". Yet, despite a move to the "quiet of Queens", my parents' marriage wouldn't make it past my second birthday, which left me as another 1980s kid living with divorce. Luckily for me, though, it happened before I can remember, and the lack of memories that I have of my parents together made them being apart just my normal. Nonetheless, having two homes would eventually get complicated—especially as an undiagnosed Autistic kid.

For my first five years on this planet, my differences were written off as adorable quirks. I began reading and speaking very early, a hyperverbal hyperlexic they call it, which was always met with delight by adults. "Oh look how smart she is!" "She is reading such a big book!" "She uses such big words!" "She is so advanced", well-meaning adults would coo. I had even potty-trained myself unprompted. But at the same time as folks were saying all of those things, my mom wrote this in my baby book about four-year-old me: "She may be intellectually gifted, but she is also emotionally stunted."

Sure, my interests were odd for a little girl as I preferred quietly digging in the mud and reading to playing with others. And yes, mealtimes, bathing, and dressing were fraught with anxiety and tears, but I was walking and talking on time, so all must be well. Such was the thinking of the world around me.

But at five, school begins to enter the picture and with it comes comparison. Suddenly surrounded by peers, it became clear that I was different. And, for the first time, I began to feel different.

Having to attend school meant uncomfortable clothes, not doing as I pleased, and having to stay someplace even if it smelled funny, was too bright, or too loud. Even if I had to keep my shoes on. I struggled with being without my mom, which meant her leaving me every day was a traumatic event for both of us.

On weekends, I had to pack all of my favorite things and head to my dad's apartment. He had returned to closer to the Bronx and was living in Yonkers. These weekend expeditions meant hours in the car both ways. It meant crossing two bridges, three tolls, and the endless honking of NYC traffic. These weekends also meant packing, and unpacking, all the things I could possibly need or want for two days because my dad's house was nothing like my mom's. I'm sure many kids of divorce found having two of everything fun, loved their time in the car with one parent or the other, and never gave packing a second thought, but for an unidentified little me, it was nothing short of torture; a torture I would request an end to, and be denied, at 12 years old.

At 12, I would experience my first Autistic burnout. It was triggered by the growing social expectations of that age, aka girls are so mean, and my first big transition, the move to middle school. But I was not diagnosed, and it was not called burnout, it was called "being difficult". I wasn't afforded the kind of recovery Autistics require and was instead sent to try one school after another. Some were so far from home, I had to use the NYC bus system, alone. Others were designed for "troubled kids" and other school refusers like me. None of them addressed my needs.

I ended up missing most of seventh and eighth grade. In an act of sheer desperation, my mother sent me to my dad's to go to school where he now lived in New Jersey. A smart choice on her part, as school was more comfortable than his house for me, but with that my entire world turned upside down. I was exhausted, angry, depressed, and defeated, but I was once again attending school. With my weekend trips reversed, I headed home to Queens on the weekends and eventually graduated high school and headed to college right on time at 18.

When my mom apologized for not doing better, my first thought was about all the times she must be thinking about. All the family holidays she had to make excuses for, all the times she had to go to work and leave me crying, all the times she needed a parenting partner and didn't have one, all the times she had to make painful choices because she thought it was the best option. All of the times that she hoped she was the best parent she could be. In all of the moments, she could have used some guidance or some perspective, or even just some community, but quite literally the information wasn't available and there wasn't anybody to ask.

Today there is somebody to ask. There are lots of somebodies, in fact! As a dedicated advocate for our community, I end up being a resource for lots of parents like my mom. One of those moms, Penny, could be my mom. She is a single mother of an only Autistic daughter who is working her behind off to support them both. They live in Brooklyn. She is busy and stressed but also loves her daughter above all else, exactly the way she is.

Penny just wants to be the best mom she can be every single day. She has tried to learn all that she can about autism but doesn't have a ton of spare time or energy to vet what she is reading or to stay current. She tries to be patient and kind with her daughter but also finds herself frustrated with her own lack of knowledge. She feels like she is constantly putting out fires in front of her, so she cannot plan for future calm. In hopes of finding out all the right answers to her questions, Penny reached out to me.

What my mom wanted at that moment was somebody to tell her exactly what she should have done and to explain exactly why she needed to do those things. Penny is in search of this knowledge too, and she's not alone. This book is my answer to Penny, to all of the Pennys, and most importantly, it is the answer I wasn't able to give my mom on that sunny evening in May. It's a journey through my life, offering insights into the Autistic experience, practical advice, and, above all, the understanding that you're not alone in this. We may not have all the answers, but together we can find a way to embrace, support, and celebrate our Autistic children for the unique individuals they are.

2
Cat lover

For as long as I can remember I have been a cat-nip-carrying ailurophile, or lover of cats. Those feisty felines captured my attention before I could walk and I continue to obsess about their perfect little toeses and noses, their tornado-of-knives fearlessness, and their elegant aloofness to this day. They are such a big part of my life that as I type this, one of my six current cats is by my side with his paw on my hand ensuring that he makes these pages. Well there, Miller, my greeter cat, kitchen troll, and fabulous house panther, the folks reading know you left your pawprint on these pages.

My love of cats has also influenced how I function in the world. Watching cat behavior has taught me endless adulting skills and how to clearly express my needs. For example, cats showed me how to conserve my energy while still being alert, how to read body language better and faster to avoid consequences, and how to be clever, resilient, and brave in the face of anything bigger than you. In turn, I have learned A LOT about cats, spending decades deep-diving into all I can to understand them back. I spent decades learning about tail flicks, vocal range, and purr frequencies, and in return, I have had the pleasure of sharing my entire existence on this planet with cats. Seriously, I have NEVER lived without a cat.

Luckily, a little girl who loves cats never really sets off alarm bells. And even though I knew my love of animals was different and bigger than anyone else's, the response from the outside world was nothing but a nod and a smile. As far as Autistic special interests go, cats were safe. But when I began demanding enough glow-in-the-dark stars to replicate the northern hemisphere on my bedroom ceiling, eyebrows began to raise. When I moved away from memorizing dinosaur names to reading about anthropologic expeditions and fossil recovery, those eyebrows turned to stares. And, while other girls my age were collecting Barbies and Cabbage Patch Dolls, I was busy researching the tectonic plates and trying to understand how volcanoes get created. But what finally raised those red flags, and brought in the special interest police, was my unwavering interest in true crime, in particular, serial killers.

I honestly have no exact memory of how I got interested in serial killers, but if I had to venture a guess, anthropology led to psychology, which led to abnormal psychology. In other words, I was attracted to the outliers like me, those that were internally different but fit right in on the outside, until they didn't. Ted Bundy, Jeffrey Dahmer, and Ed Kemper, for example. I was fascinated by what made them tick and even more interested in the way so many of them were brilliantly deranged and living two lives. I guess I found the parallels to my reality as intriguing as they were disturbing.

In any case, by high school, I was fully engaged in this topic. I had read all of the books available to me, memorized a ton of facts, and even picked my favorite killers. So, when a history teacher asked for a report related to our unit about the 1960s, it took me all of two seconds to choose Charles Manson and his gaggle of girls. Needless to say, though he was a valid choice for the period, Charlie and I did not find a fan in my teacher and my guidance counselor was notified.

Since I was a relatively good, if rebellious, student, I was sent off in confusion with a warning to watch my topics of interest. Nobody cared how excited I was to put the report together. Nobody cared about my attention to detail or skill with the written word. Nobody even acknowledged my perfect grammar. All they did was point out that what I found interesting, and was good at, was not okay, and I needed to change. It was not unlike all the other times when I was younger and would get excited about something, like tectonic plates, and folks would criticize my volume or flappy hands, very literally correcting my joy.

Cats, tectonic plates, and serial killers were all what we Autistic people now call SPINS or special interests. Some of you may be familiar enough with Autistics to spot a SPIN or an info dump when you see one, while others may not yet have the vocabulary to describe it. For many of us—especially as kids but even into adulthood—our SPINs are used against us, and our deep interest in a certain, very specific something sets us apart and leads to us frequently being called "weird". This is why many of us hesitate to share our SPINs.

Early work on autism discouraged SPINs, seeing them as yet another thing that makes us different, another thing to get rid of, and that is exactly what they taught our families to do. Parents followed this misguided advice and began to use their children's SPINs as part of a reward and punishment system.

For Autistics, a special interest, or SPIN, is an area of intense focus, interest, and knowledge, while also being an essential component of our quality of life (Grove et al., 2018). Autistics usually spend a good deal of our time (and brain space) on our SPINs, and we often feel emotionally attached to them in much the same way non-Autistics feel attached to family members, some of which they don't know well or see often. In addition, Autistics often feel so attached to our SPINS that there is a period of grief, much like losing a loved one, when we move on from one. It is super important that people understand that SPINs are necessary and valuable to Autistics and should not ever be minimized as an "intense hobby".

Sometimes our SPINs are lifelong, like my reverence for felines, while other times, one will slowly extinguish and we wait, in grief and dysregulation, for another to ignite. Some of us boast a library of interests, while others of us only require one or two at a time. For most of us, the pursuit of our interests is a private event that is often done in "hyper-focus mode", which is our way of decompressing, turning off the world, and regulating ourselves.

Our SPINs are a necessity, not an indulgence. We don't just want them; we NEED them to regulate and thrive. Studies carried out in the last 15 years are validating what many Autistics have always known: apart from their potential to establish a profession, they consistently boost self-esteem and assist individuals in managing their emotions. Research indicates that they may also aid in the socialization and education of Autistic kids (Kapp et al., 2013; Milton, 2012). Special interests are beginning to be embraced by educators and physicians rather than being suppressed or erased. Teachers are incorporating them into their lesson plans.

"There's been a lot of negative language used around special interests, things like 'inflexible' and 'obsessions'", says psychologist Rachel Grove, a research fellow at the University of Technology Sydney in Australia. "The real paradigm shift is thinking about special interests as more positive" (Kapp et al., 2013).

In the book *What I Want to Talk About*, popular autism advocate Pete Wharmby takes readers on a journey through his special interests, explaining how they gave him energy and focus (Wharmby, 2022). In this book he explains that special interests are the results of monotropic focus, but that focus can lead to forgetting to eat, sleep, or use the bathroom for hours when tuned into his passion. If you love an Autistic person, it's important to know that SPINs are essential and to treat them with respect and reverence, while also bringing us a snack and reminding us to take a nap from time to time.

Fortunately (and unfortunately) for me, my mom had no information about SPINs either way. There was nobody to tell her she needed to stop me, and as a single mom in Queens, I'm sure she appreciated that I was silently, and safely, keeping myself occupied, albeit with some strange topics instead of with other kids. What she did instead is revolutionary by modern parenting standards, but she quite simply trusted her gut and supported my passions without judgment. And whatever my current enthusiasm was, it was never used as a reward or punishment for unrelated actions. Meaning that, in the confines of our home, I was allowed to pursue my interests to my heart's delight, and on most days, she would entertain me by pretending to be interested in them too. It was in those moments that I loved my mom the most. Because in those moments, I felt wholly loved and completely understood.

In addition to providing a means to regulation, Autistic SPINs feed directly into our natural strengths in both our capacity for memorizing details and our naturally sophisticated logical reasoning. And in return for our dedication, we often find ourselves experts on a huge variety of topics, starting at a very young age. Thus, lending to the colloquial term for young Autistics like me, twice exceptional.

3
Twice exceptional

Before identifying as Autistic, I identified as an Information Seeker. My brain is simply happiest when it is drowned in new data, and as such, I am happiest when learning something new or layering deeper knowledge onto an existing base. And for as long as I can remember, my motivation for doing anything has always been to understand all that I can about everything that I can. This has also always meant that the most frequently used word in my vocabulary is "why".

While in general being a curious child is often met with positivity, in the pre-Google world, my preoccupation with why was as much of a nuisance as it was something to marvel at. Because, of course, once my singular focus was drawn to a topic, it would mean unending hours of me talking endlessly about everything I learned along the way; the classic Autistic info dump.

By about six or seven years old, thanks to my very own complete World Book encyclopedia set, my interest had moved from baby animals to volcanoes. With nobody else to share the learning burden, at some point my poor mom had heard enough about the difference between lava and magma and sent me back to my room, my very favorite place to be. My room was my sanctuary. It was where I carefully displayed that World Book and the giant dictionaries that went with it. It was where I lined up all my furry plush toys and hid all the hard-faced plastic dolls that dared to invade. It was where I could safely disappear into a book and the only place my brain could find silence from the cacophony that is living in NYC. And, perhaps most importantly, it was where I was most free to indulge in being my authentic Autistic self. Naturally, this had to be where I would hold my very first class on volcanoes. And let's be very clear, I felt called to teach a class, a group versus an individual.

I mean, here I was still in single digits, being rejected for my desire to pass on the information that I learned, and my response was to turn around and not only keep doing it but to do so with even more people at one time. Back then, my resilience was just beginning to show, but my innate desire to teach others would be one I would come to rely on as the foundation for my advocacy work and my career.

Each day after school, my new favorite thing to do was to create my classroom. My plush toys would make excellent students, and that would be an easy solution to filling the class. So, instead of setting them down in "seats", I began with writing and creating our textbook and eventually the workbook that went with it.

My mom would often brag to folks that I was her "Encyclopedia". At family gatherings, I would hear her proudly announce that folks could ask the "Encyclopedia". On her phone calls, I would hear her say things like, "I don't know where she gets it from, but she is a genius." And, honestly, I loved my encyclopedia, and I loved making her proud. It was pretty okay to hear my mom say with a smile, "She is just like a walking encyclopedia. She takes in everything, and she retains it all." Which was all fine and well until the "everything" I was taking in became too much.

You see, this magnificent ability to take in all the details had some unfortunate side effects. To begin with, overwhelm is never too far away. It feels like my brain is always collecting information from around me, but it is unable to sift through and decide what is most important. Instead, it takes in all the details as though they are equally important. So, while some folks can be in a room full of different noises, smells, and colors, and still carry on a conversation, I become so quickly overwhelmed by taking in all of the details that I often lose the ability to speak. Sometimes in these scenarios, I can maintain one- or two-word sentences, while at other times I cannot even make my lips move.

Historically, the autism spectrum has been understood as a linear continuum from "low functioning" to "high functioning". This framework utilizes functioning labels like "high-functioning autism" and "profound autism" to indicate a person's support needs and capacities as perceived by the observer. However, our ability to function is something that fluctuates. It tends to ebb and flow throughout the course of our lives, often changing from year to year, if not day to day, as a result of how especially complicated it can be to be an Autistic in today's world.

Because of these fixed, and often not so helpful or accurate functioning labels, my autism went unrecognized and my need for support in these areas also went unrecognized, as I masked distress behind academic achievement. The resulting trauma still impacts me decades later.

What my experience with twice exceptionality and my reputation as the Encyclopedia taught me was that there is a danger in thinking that Autistic people like me can appear like we don't need a lot of supports to function. My mom was doing her best to support me by bragging about my strengths, but what that encouraged me to cover up were the areas where I did need help as they were what was leading to situational mutism, exhaustion, shut-down, and burnout at the early age of 12.

It is essential that we understand that static and linear functioning labels are not helpful in accommodating our fluctuating needs. When we use functioning labels, we minimize the internal realities and unseen vulnerabilities of so-called "high-functioning" Autistics. The intense world theory helps explain why. Many Autistics sense stimuli more acutely than the neuromajority, while simultaneously missing the innate ability to filter inputs and edit responses. As a result, those of us with high aptitudes in some areas, like data collection and pattern recognition, may also experience debilitating repercussions from sensory overload, chronic pain and physical exhaustion, and co-occurring mental health issues. Brilliance in one area often coincides with extensive support needs in others, with the former, in some cases, eclipsing the latter to the detriment of the Autistic person themselves.

So, not only were my needs being missed and not met, but I was learning that my value and worth very much relied upon my twice exceptionality. I got so much positive reinforcement for these aspects of who I was that I began to act this way even when I didn't feel this way. This inauthentic persona is what we call masking, and it is an unsustainable, trauma-induced, coping mechanism that leads directly to struggles like mutism, chronic pain, and sometimes, even, burnout, or worse. Autistic masking involves hiding aspects of one's social, sensory, cognitive, or behavioral responses to fit in or avoid stigma, either consciously or unconsciously. A study found that both Autistic and non-Autistic people reported exhaustion and unhappiness due to masking, feeling disconnected from their true identity. However, some aspects were more specific to Autistic individuals, such as sensory suppression and masking leading to suicidal ideation (Miller, Rees, and Pearson, 2021; Pearson and Rose, 2021).

It's hard to remember the first time I became situationally mute, but what I do remember is that it happened so often that it was remarked upon. At home, I was notorious for talking nonstop. Motormouth was a term my close family used often. But, outside of our tiny bubble, the words would disappear, getting harder to reach the louder, bigger, smellier the here and now was and the longer we were out in it. In those moments, whether it be social or sensory overload or both, I felt trapped. A frightened brain trapped in a frozen body, too immature to identify my needs, and too overwhelmed to get them met anyway.

When aspects of cognition come easily, other developmental domains often lag behind. For example, while I had advanced reading ability, I also had motoric delays causing clumsiness. I learned to rely heavily on my intellectual strengths to mask social communication differences, but during the inevitable dips in functioning, my mask would slip, revealing support gaps like my situational mutism that sadly were missed.

These multidimensional trade-offs illustrate why the spectrum metaphor proves misleading. Autism is perhaps better visualized as a pizza pie with skills, aptitudes, and support needs as slices rather than placed on a straight line. Each hand-cut slice is a slightly different size than the one next to it and gets its own amount of toppings. Some slices get full of toppings; other slices look a little empty. Someone requiring significant personal assistance due to chronic illness or motor issues may have intellectual gifts enabling self-advocacy, while a socially outgoing Autistic could still collapse into overload meltdowns without timely sensory respite. And each day we are presented with the challenge to make the pizza we can with ingredients we have on hand at that specific time.

Crucially, the fluctuating nature of functioning means yesterday's "high-functioning" presentation provides little insight into today or tomorrow's support necessities. For example, I may articulate complex ideas through writing, yet struggle to make a simple phone call to cancel an appointment during periods of executive functioning lapses or mental exhaustion. An intellectually gifted child could lose critical services after hitting arbitrary metrics of "success" that fail to reflect their lived experience. This pressure to constantly perform at narrow definitions of high achievement can exacerbate distress and create trauma. Judgments by functioning often become weapons wielded against support needs in the war for quality of life.

For decades, I was all but silent outside of our first-floor apartment and a few other choice locations like my grandparents' houses and a few neighbors. I was either busy being brilliant or stubbornly sitting in a corner, still and expressionless, face in a book or staring off lost in thought. And rarely, if ever, would I be found with friends or other kids at all.

While I didn't have the term for it at the time, I had special needs in two ways: I needed more support and help in some areas, and I needed space to excel in others. I was, in fact, twice exceptional— at the top and the bottom of some system of standards that was in no way standard to me. Twice exceptional students possess both extraordinary gifts and disabilities. In my school years, however, I was considered so gifted that I deserved or earned extra resources from the school. "Lucky" (or maybe not so lucky) for me, I was talented enough at masking my disabilities that I was tapped to be among the "Gifted and Talented" students.

My mom wanted me to be happy, and when I was accepted into the Gifted and Talented program this seemed like the answer to a prayer. Here my brilliance would be fully celebrated. I was happy to be recognized too, and even more happy to leave regular classes to participate. But I think part of me had a hunch that there was a dark side of being labeled "gifted", which was the way that it cemented the idea that my value came from my intelligence. So, when I struggled with something, like math, due to my unrecognized dyscalculia, I began to feel like an imposter and my self-esteem began to shrink. Dyscalculia causes challenges such as difficulties with numbers, trouble differentiating mathematical signs, and challenges in conceptualizing time. It also delves into the potential causes of those challenges, including neurological factors and deficits in working memory (Intriago, Rodríguez, and Cevallos, 2021).

These tensions between strength and disability figure prominently in debates around twice exceptionality. Gifted and talented programs arose in schools during the 1980s to nurture standout intellectual, creative, and academic ability. However, admission often relied on narrow definitions of accomplishment. Spaces just didn't seem to exist for my asynchronous development, leading me to believe spaces didn't exist for me.

As the neurodiversity movement has grown, so has the idea of "twice exceptional students". The quest is no longer to get the smart kids to perform at their maximum ability but to equip them with tools to fulfill their talent without burning out.

Progress comes from drawing connections between the strengths and barriers facing gifted and disabled students. With responsive instruction adapting to learning variability, twice exceptional children can thrive. Their regulation issues can be eased through accommodations like flexible deadlines and sensory-friendly classrooms, which were never even considered when I was coming of age. It almost seems like the gifted and talented programs I was in were designed to speed up depression, anxiety, and burnout!

Rather than view disability and giftedness as contradictory, modern frameworks see them as complex intersections deserving personalized support. The one question my mom wanted answered above all others was, "How can such a 'smart kid' struggle so much?" The short answer to that question is that my Autistic brain was, and still is, at odds with the world around me most of the time, especially when it came to both my sensory and social differences.

Moving beyond static and linear functioning labels makes space for flexible thinking, planning, and support accommodations. Instead of classifying individual competence, the priority becomes identifying each Autistic person's customized array of strengths, talents, resources, and barriers in a variety of areas. From there, advocates can help establish individual support strategies for empowering self-determination and dignity.

We all have periods of high performance as well as lows. For Autistics, though, the pendulum often swings much farther and faster in both directions. Without the right supports, the lows can be extremely isolating and dangerously dark places masking significant trauma that lingers for decades.

All any of us truly want is to be empowered and accepted for who we really are under the surface—even when society sees only where we fall short. Progress and inclusion will come when we embrace all minds and abilities and accommodations that empower each of us to reach our full potential, and that manifest uniquely in strengths, passions, and purpose over a lifetime.

I share my story in hopes the next generation will inherit a more inclusive world, where their gifts can soar without shame or secrecy, or the need to sacrifice health or hide hardship to justify respect and dignity. But the one place many Autistics, like me, have always felt respected and safe—perhaps since the Ptolemaic Dynasty of Egypt way back in 300 or so BCE—is the library. Because if Autistic people are unified about anything, it's our love for that magical institution.

4
Library kid

On the day I found it I could not wait to get home from the library. It was a fairly new paperback for our small Queens, NY branch, but the cover made it clear that many before me had already read and enjoyed this book. That day it was my turn.

I flew past that cover and all the other nonsense they put before the actual book begins and settled in for a great read, which opened with the line, "The naked child ran out of the hide-covered lean-to toward the rocky beach at the bend in the small river. It didn't occur to her to look back. Nothing in her experience ever gave her reason to doubt the shelter and those within it would be there when she returned" (Auel, 2002).

Already a keen reader of all things anthropology and archeology, at age eight I discovered memoirs, biographies, and something called historical fiction. *Clan of the Cave Bear* was a long book, my favorite kind, which is part of why I picked it up. The other reason was that there was a second book coming out related to this one and a good series was, and is, one of my very favorite things. I mean, if I am going to lose myself somewhere interesting, I'd like to be lost there for a while. This series was about a little pre-historic orphan girl growing up just after the last glacial period of the current ice age had occurred, and it already had me hooked.

I read as much as I could that night and, naturally, brought the book with me to school the next day.

It was right about here that my love for reading got me in trouble for the first time. Up until that point, I was nothing but commended for reading books at an adult level. Grown-ups couldn't believe that I was browsing in their section of the library, always nodding with pride at my choices. Having earned the right to read books from home if I finished my second-grade required reading, I chose to breeze through the year's worth of classroom reading assignments quickly, leaving me reading my own books by October. And on that fateful post-October day, I pulled my new, long book out of my Garfield backpack to pick up where I left off. I didn't understand everything I was reading but it was fascinating to read about how these Cro-Magnon and Neanderthal clans lived.

The details of what followed are fuzzy around the edges all these years later, but I know my teacher took my book. My next report card had a note about "reading material not suitable for the classroom". And though I don't remember how far into the book I got, I had apparently read enough that my mom and I had to have our first sex talk. To this day I am not positive that I ever finished that book, nor have I ever seen the second one, but I have heard the series did quite well with a group that was obviously not supposed to be made up of eight-year-old girls hyper-focused on human evolution.

Thankfully, this incident didn't deter me from reading. It just taught me how to be more particular with my material. As a city kid, I had the entire New York City Public Library system one librarian request away. Our branch itself was quite small, but if the book was in the system at any branch, even the big Manhattan ones, my librarian could ask for it to be sent right to us for free with my valid library card. I loved our little branch for how quiet it was most of the time and, since it was right next to my school, it was where I waited when I got out of class for my mom to get off work and pick me up.

In the time before we were all "connected", books were my cell phone. I would lug whatever I was currently reading around with me everywhere. And any time the world became too much or too boring, I could disappear into those pages and find regulation. And much the way parents consider screen time with their kids today is how my mom felt about my reading way back then. While most people remarked on how cute it was that I "always had my nose in a book" and how quietly I "kept myself occupied", I could see how they judged me every time I pulled out a book at a family event or in a restaurant.

Books, and later music and movies, are the best and most reliable way for me to stay regulated. I didn't understand back then but I spent my first three decades on this planet feeling overwhelmed and seeking approval for the calm, alone time that so many Autistics seem to require. What my mom didn't understand, and what others were judging, was that my response to the instinct to protect my overwhelmed brain was to shut down and read. It was the only way I knew to regulate myself. There were no stim toys and fidgets. Nobody was encouraging me to get up and take a walk. And one can only escape to the bathroom so many times.

Self-regulation plays an essential role in our communication, our well-being, and our ability to thrive, but for Autistic people, finding regulation can be a daily struggle. Whether or not you have New York City as a backdrop, we live in a loud world and we all must find ways to regulate. For me, I found regulation by giving into my love of information seeking. I knew if I had a book with me, it would all be okay. That I had an escape route; a way to stop the pot from boiling over.

My mom seemed to understand that I needed my books. As a heavy reader herself, it seemed to be something she could kind of understand. Something she could get behind enough to defend me against the judgmental looks from family members. Of course, not all Autistics find regulation at our local library. Many of us find regulation from spinning or flapping. Still others feel best when swimming or running. Some of us carry fidgets and some of us wear compression clothes. Whatever the tactic, the end goal is the same: regulation.

My voracious reading and the ability to self-regulate came as a result of my natural strength with words being nurtured, praised, and encouraged. The same could not be said in the realm of numbers. While college-level reading came to me with ease, once my math class moved from basic arithmetic to fractions, it all went blurry, in a very literal sense.

Unbeknown to all involved, me included, I have a learning disability related to numbers called dyscalculia. It's not surprising I spent most of my life without that knowledge. In context, it was the 1980s and I was one of the too many shoved into our NYC public school system. And in that system, you were either gifted in all areas, or not gifted at all. Convinced I was being stubborn and refusing to do math, the praises for my reading silenced in favor of endless hours of focus on the thing I struggled with the most. It was impossible by the standards back then for me to be so comprehensive verbally yet so unable to achieve that level when numerical concepts were involved. All of the focus suddenly on my weaknesses led quickly to low self-esteem.

Many Autistics have what is known as a "spiky profile". That refers to the way that some Autistic individuals will excel in certain areas or with certain tasks but struggle in others (Wilson, 2023). In other words, Autistics not only exhibit a wide range of strengths and weaknesses, but there is usually a large disparity between those strengths and weaknesses—for example, my hyperlexia (the ability to read at levels far beyond those expected for their age) versus my dyscalculia (the IN-ability to handle math- and number-related tasks). Having a spiky profile means when I understand something I understand it better than most, but when I miss something, I REALLY miss it. But that's a story for the next chapter.

What's important to take away from the spiky profile is that there is no "normal" for Autistic development. We each get our own personal brand of autism and the strengths and challenges that come with it. It really is that simple. We are never going to sit neatly in the middle of a bell curve. When assessing your child's development, focus on nurturing their self-esteem, focus on encouraging their unique strengths. This will help you and them to recognize their innate value while also fostering a sense of pride in their abilities. However, it is crucial to balance this with the insights from Chapter 3 on avoiding burnout. While encouraging their talents, make sure you are attentive to signs of stress or fatigue. Ensure they have ample time to recharge, to experience joy, and to simply be their authentic Autistic selves. This balanced approach promotes individual development, while valuing them for who they are and not just for their accomplishments. By observing their behavior and listening to their needs, you can provide a supportive environment that cultivates their self-esteem while safeguarding their well-being.

An entry by my mom in my baby book references my spiky profile. She writes in an entry from before I was four years old, "She is intellectually advanced but emotionally stunted." Pretty darn close, no? I remember it was painful to read those words post diagnosis because of their accuracy. It made me sad to know my differences were apparent from so early on and yet it took decades to be identified.

My mother's observation in my baby book was an early recognition of this spiky profile—a term that aptly describes the divergent paths of development in Autistic individuals. Her words, "intellectually advanced but emotionally stunted", although stark, were a prescient reflection of the complexities I would navigate throughout my life.

This realization, though painful in its accuracy, also brought a sense of clarity. It underscored the importance of early recognition and support for Autistic individuals. Understanding that these early signs are not just quirks but indicators of a deeper, intrinsic wiring can change the trajectory of an Autistic child's life.

It can lead to more tailored support, greater acceptance, and a deeper appreciation of their unique capabilities.

For parents like my mother, grappling with the enigma of an Autistic child, this story serves as a reminder of the critical role of observation, understanding, and support. It's essential to recognize and celebrate the strengths while patiently navigating the challenges. By doing so, you not only affirm the value of your child's uniquely wired brain but also foster an environment where they can truly thrive.

5
Autistic naivety

The thing about having a brain that does things differently than most brains is that you have no idea until someone points it out. As the proud owner of a different brain, I can tell you that, most of the time, I am baffled by the way that the neurotypical brain works. I can also tell you that neurotypicals tend to feel the same way about me and my brain. It took me decades, and a late-in-life autism diagnosis, to be able to look back at the early misunderstandings with any amount of humor, but I finally can.

I learned early on that being grown-up means "doing errands". Being raised by a single, working mom, it was one of the first things about adulthood that I was certain about. Errands like grocery shopping, taking the car "in", and stopping at the bank are boring things that must get done in order for you to do anything fun. On any given day, my mom would check the running list of errands in her brain she kept for us to complete when she wasn't at work. And we always had to do those things first, before any kind of joy, so that is what I figured being an adult would mean.

On one of our regular after-work and school errand runs, we were headed to the bank. Back then, if you had any banking to do, it meant a trip in the car to wait in a long line to talk to a person who apparently controlled the money and your access to it. There was nothing about the bank or money that I found interesting. It was an almost windowless building that somehow managed to smell like a combination of freshly made photocopies and a dentist's waiting room. The air lightly filled with vague, mellow, instrumental music and the smell of mixed perfumes and hot ink. Clean but utilitarian is bank couture and it's certainly a place where time stands still, and sunshine is replaced with fluorescent overhead lighting.

So, when an orange awning appeared to signify that the drive-thru window that was added to our otherwise boring, gray, stucco-covered box of a bank was open for business it was incredibly exciting, to say the least. Finally, there was an errand that I could get behind. If riding through the car wash was cool, how cool would seeing behind the bank counter be? And without having to leave the comfort of our little gray Volkswagen Jetta? Count me in!

As we made our way to the bank drive-thru for the first time, I was excited enough to be wiggly in my seat. So, when my mom pulled over before we got there, I was a little surprised and asked her why. She explained that we would need to wait until the next day to go because her paycheck wouldn't clear for another day. Confused, and pretty disappointed by the unplanned delay in our plans, I needed more information quickly. What did her paycheck have to do with the bank? I figured maybe she didn't understand how it worked and slowly explained that the drive-thru worked just like the regular bank. We could just drive up like we walk in and ask for our money like we normally do. It wasn't that complicated. The bank is where you get money from, right?

You see, in my head, the bank, like all other "errands", was just another boring store we had to go to before we could go to the park or get McDonald's. You go to the grocery store for food, the gas station for gas, and the bank for money. That simple. The concept that you had to put money into the bank for it to be there for taking out just did not exist for me. Nor did the concept that you had to work to earn a paycheck to get the money that you put in the bank.

Since nobody had taken the time to teach me all the steps that revolve around money, I didn't understand the connection between work and money, and I didn't understand that money had to be earned, that it wasn't just given to you when you pull up to the drive-thru as an adult.

My mom was deeply amused by my confusion; she laughed a lot in the car and repeated the story for many years to come to amuse others. But what she never shared with others was the recognition at that moment that maybe my encyclopedic talents weren't the only different thing about me. Because, though I could retain endless amounts of data, I was obviously missing other things that most of my peers already understood, but she couldn't understand why.

The Autistic brain does not glean information from the world around us in the same way. Today I would explain it as Autistics learn by doing but not by observation alone. Meaning, that our brains do not absorb information simply by being in the vicinity of it; we need to be doing it, and often multiple times, before our brains latch on. But when we get it, it never leaves. So, while other kids were gathering information about the world bit by bit simply by exposure, my brain was only paying attention to what I was interested in and what I needed to do. It makes me think of all the college students who leave for school but don't know how to do their laundry. Most of them understand the concept of laundry, and many can even vaguely tell you the steps, but when it comes down to getting it done, it becomes clear that they have never actually done a single load. It's a form of learned helplessness that occurs all too frequently to Autistics. If you are not the owner of an Autistic brain, it can be easy to assume that we simply cannot do something, rather than to pause and wonder if we are being taught the information in a modality that works for us. Often this presumed incompetence translates into well-meaning folks doing too many things for us, instead of taking the time to do things WITH us, and that's where we start to get lost. Autistics can't know what we are capable of unless we get the chance to try and do it ourselves.

Errands were a constant source of these kinds of stories. It was when my mom and I would spend the most time together, and it was also the time I felt most comfortable asking questions. Since I was a kid who could name over 50 cat breeds, my mom assumed I knew more about the way the world worked than I actually did, and since my intelligence was directly tied to my value, I didn't ask questions often. Instead, my info-seeking brain would research, and the answers, like the questions, were for me alone. Questions I had learned over time, especially about regular everyday things, were not interesting to me and also usually exposed that I wasn't as smart as everyone kept saying.

One such question surrounded the origins of the endless pints, quarts, and gallons of cold, white milk filling the dairy aisle of our local grocery store. There was always so much of it and it came in so many sizes by so many companies, but for the life of me, I could not figure out how all this milk got made and then why it came so many different ways. So, one day, I decided it was time to ask out loud. As we made our way past the rows and rows of the white stuff, I turned to my mom and asked, "How do they make milk?" To which my mom replied, "Ask the cows."

"What? Do cows speak? How can I ask them?" I thought.

After a few more clarifying questions, I was horrified to find out that the milk in the containers at the grocery store wasn't a manufactured beverage like iced tea or fruit punch but was in fact the exact same milk that baby cows drink. So weird and gross! My mom was equally horrified that her encyclopedia of a daughter, who loved animals, had so innocently assumed that milk was a human invention. But there we were, me no longer a milk drinker, and my mom, baffled and without guidance.

Unfortunately, in a world created by the neuromajority, clarifying questions can often be a trap. In adulthood, Autistic communication continues to be misunderstood. Our directness is seen as rude, our passion is seen as "too much", and our honesty is seen as a weakness. But what makes us feel the most gaslit is when our clarifying queries are misinterpreted as "questioning authority". And it happens all the time.

According to my best comprehension of the social expectations of the neuromajority, clarifying questions are seen as a direct challenge to authority. While Autistics are simply requesting further information or context, our asks are too often received as something more sinister.

Though Autistics are often told we are terrible at communication, what folks really mean is that we are terrible at non-Autistic communication. Despite the fact that clarifying questions are necessary for good communication, out in the world our questions are most often misinterpreted or dismissed entirely, while we are doing our best to make sure we have understood the assignment at hand.

The first time I remember experiencing this was way back in the first grade. Mrs Plotznick was my teacher, and she was a character! One of the ways I survived school was by hyper-focusing on my teachers. I found the details of their clothes, the way they walked, and how they spoke fascinating. Mrs Plotznick did not disappoint. She was a short lady somewhere in her 60s who imagined herself a fancy art museum Manhattanite despite spending five days a week in a crappy public elementary school in Queens. Her outfits were always a little out there, bright, and big, not like the other teachers in their drab turtlenecks and pencil skirts. Her hair was equally a marvel, teased, bleach blonde, and pinned up with something artsy, though the amount of hairspray she used did the job by itself. Below the massive blonde head, she painted on big makeup with loud eyeshadow and too much orange-red lipstick. She smelled like Aqua Net hairspray and baby powder, and I was hypnotized by her.

We knew as a class that she loved art and so it was usually a low-pressure part of our week when she would declare it was time for art. I am a creative person by nature, but not a particularly artistic one, yet I was all about art time. To me it represented quiet time in our classroom where I was actually encouraged to spend time with my thoughts and ideas. For me, the only time at school that I liked better than art was when we went lights out for movie time.

On one particular day, art time was declared, and we were given an assignment: draw a face. Faces weren't something I really liked. Eyes can be creepy and mouths gross. Still, it was art and that meant freedom, right? Freedom to choose any color you could imagine and faces that came in all sizes, shapes, and combinations. So, I grabbed my crayons and got to business. I made a purple circle with orange cat ears, one giant green eye, no nose or mouth but a solid set of black whiskers, and a big head of curly, blue hair. A magnificent, creative, and wholly unique approach to faces! Great job, me.

Or not so great job, according to good ol' Mrs Plotznick.

As she made her way around the room looking over shoulders and above heads at each carefully drawn face, she would nod in approval or ooh or aah as she took in the talents of a room of restless seven-year-olds. When she got to my desk, she leaned over my shoulder to inspect my art and sighed. Not the sigh of someone who has experienced true creativity for the first time, but more like someone who has found themselves stuck in bumper-to-bumper traffic on the Grand Central Parkway for the gazillionth day in a row. It was the kind of sigh I would get used to hearing from the adults around me who were not as amused by my differences as my mom was.

"That is not a face. I asked you to draw a face. Faces have two eyes, two ears, a triangle nose, and a round mouth", and she went to the board and drew it. Well, I was pretty sure she didn't give us those rules at the beginning of art and I was also pretty sure that art was one of those things that didn't come in right and wrong. Confused, I needed more information, so I braved a question.

"Isn't art about interpretation?", my seven-year-old self asked. I mean, that's what all the archaeology books said about the profiles of the Egyptians found on the pyramids. And those faces didn't all have two eyes, two ears, a mouth, and a nose. In fact, some of that art, like the Sphinx, was just like my face, a mix of species. And with that, I found myself sitting in the principal's office listening to phones ring until art was over.

This is when I started getting labeled. I would become a frequent visitor to the office in the years to come and eventually would be a regular in "class" with our guidance counselor, too. My report cards started including words like difficult, over-emotional, dramatic, stubborn, and, somehow, lazy. After that, I was never called a different thinker, nor were any of my strengths ever recognized, and I could no longer relish in the comfort that I was the "smart kid". Both directly and indirectly, I began to believe the descriptors being given to me and any self-esteem I had would disappear for decades. I was no longer the smart kid; I had become the "troubled kid".

The struggle in this scenario begins with something known as theory of mind. Theory of mind is a fundamental concept in psychology and cognitive science that refers to our ability to designate mental states, such as beliefs, intents, desires, emotions, knowledge, to ourselves and others, as well as our ability to understand that others have beliefs, desires, and perspectives that are different from our own (Baron-Cohen, Leslie, and Frith, 1985). This ability enables us to predict and interpret the behavior of others, understand that others have their own thoughts and feelings, and engage in complex communication and emotion like empathy. As we learn theory of mind, we get better at recognizing ourselves as individuals with distinct thoughts and feelings, separate and often different from others.

For many decades, it was believed that Autistics did not experience theory of mind and thus lacked empathy. Quite a sweeping statement and one that comes from the idea that there is only one right way to be and think. It is also completely inaccurate. In fact, most Autistics report being overly empathic, which can be overwhelming itself and lead to social communication challenges.

In response to the inaccuracy of theory of mind, psychologist Damian Milton introduced the double empathy problem, a concept that redefines our understanding of social interactions between Autistic and non-Autistic people. The double empathy problem challenges the traditional view that Autistic individuals lack empathy, instead positing that there is a mutual misunderstanding at work here (Milton, 2012). That, in fact, both Autistic and non-Autistic people struggle to empathize with each other's distinctly different way of experiencing the world. This double whammy of miscommunication comes from our differing ways of perceiving the world, with emphasis on the idea that empathy is not a universal human experience but rather influenced by our life experiences.

And influenced by life experiences I was. I'm pretty sure that my internal belief that I am bad with money started on that fateful day when my mom's paycheck was delayed. I also know for sure that I haven't had a glass of milk since I found out how it's "made". And I am fairly certain that the reason I stayed a creative person but never felt drawn to art was all thanks to my first-grade teacher.

Reflecting on these early experiences, it becomes evident that my Autistic naivety was not just a lack of understanding but a different way of interpreting the world. The confusion at the bank, the disillusionment about milk, and the confrontation over my interpretation of art in school—each of these incidents were pivotal moments in my journey of self-awareness. They were not just simple misunderstandings but profound insights into the unique workings of my Autistic mind.

These experiences highlight the critical importance of nurturing an environment where Autistic individuals can learn and explore at their own pace, in ways that align with their unique processing style. It underscores the necessity for patience, clear communication, and the opportunity to learn by doing, rather than just observing. The world often expects Autistic individuals to adapt to its norms, but these incidents show the need for a reciprocal understanding—an acknowledgment that the Autistic ways of perceiving and interacting with the world are equally valid.

Understanding that Autistic children often require explicit explanations and firsthand experiences to grasp concepts is crucial. It's not just about answering their questions; it's about recognizing that their ways of processing information are different, yet entirely valid. It's about taking those extra moments to explain the why and how, not just the what. This approach fosters an environment of trust and understanding, where your child feels valued and supported in their learning journey.

For parents, this journey with your Autistic child is not just about guiding them through the neurotypical world but also about learning from them and appreciating their perspective. It's a journey of mutual growth and understanding, where each experience, each question, each unique way of seeing the world enriches your family life. Remember, your child's Autistic mind is a wellspring of potential, creativity, and insight. By nurturing this potential, you're not just supporting your child; you're celebrating their unique contribution to the tapestry of human experience.

Embracing this perspective transforms the way we approach Autistic naivety. It's not a barrier but an opportunity—an opportunity to teach, to learn, and to grow together. It's about bridging the gap of understanding and empathy, recognizing that diversity in thought and perspective enriches our collective human experience. A component of all these experiences, and the endless others I survived, is that they have taught me to adjust my expectations when it comes to other humans, and that the more prepared I can be for any given scenario, the better my chances are of making it through it unscathed. But this is a lesson I had to learn through lots, and lots, of traumatic and formative experiences, like the ones you'll find in the next chapter.

6
Setting expectations

I don't have too many stories that involve my dad. As my parents divorced when I was so young, I spent the majority of the time with my mom, especially in my older years. I remember that I was always more comfortable being under my mom's care and that I felt really out of place when required to spend time with dad instead. He just didn't seem to get me the way that mom did and to an extent he always felt far away and like a veritable stranger. We made little effort to really get to know each other and spent our time together in the car going back and forth between houses. Leaving me with lots of memories of sitting in traffic on the Cross Bronx Expressway, passing the awkward minutes by singing along to our only shared interest, the tunes of Billy Joel, with both of us preferring his classic albums *Glass Houses* and *The Stranger*.

The rest of our weekends together, I spent wishing time would move faster so that I could go home to my room, my safe space. This feeling of being out of place with a parent is an odd one to experience and it only got more complicated when my dad married my stepmom. Nobody likes being a third wheel in someone else's relationship, but that is exactly what I ended up being. The only bonus that my stepmom came with was her funny and nurturing parental unit, my step-grandparents, I guess you would call them. Weekends with my dad were always better when we went to the apartment that my stepmother grew up in. Her parents had created the most cozy and comfortable space out of their tiny two-bedroom apartment in the Bronx. So when one weekend I was told we were headed there, I was pretty happy.

Our visits were fairly regular to their place. My dad and stepmom liked to do a lot of their errands near there, including getting haircuts. Which was fine by me as long as I got to camp out in the apartment with the comfy couches and nice assortment of snacks. On this particular day, both my dad and my stepmom were heading out to the hair place so my dad could get his biweekly cut. My dad wasn't a big man, but he was tall to me. He was somehow always just a little bit tan, with glasses, short dark hair, and a very full dark beard and mustache combo. He had maintained this look my entire life and had never deviated from it ever—until this fateful day.

My dad and stepmom had been gone for a few hours. They had walked to the haircutter who was just a short few blocks away so I knew I would see them walking up the hill if I looked out the apartment window. Sure enough, a few minutes of checking the window later, I could see their two figures walking side by side and making their way up the start of the hill. Completely unaware they were being watched, they continued to get closer and soon I was able to discern some features. As they came into focus, my heart dropped into my stomach, and I felt the blood leave my face. That man walking up the hill with my stepmom was NOT my dad. Was my stepmom having an affair?

As they got closer, I noticed the clothes and the gait of the man. "Wait," I thought, "that is my dad." But he was almost unrecognizable. He had shaved his face clean. Gone was the mustache and beard that had set my dad apart from other men, and what remained was a very smooth, very white, upper lip and chin. This man walking with my stepmom was no longer my dad.

It's taken me years to get over "the haircut". His appearance was one of the few things that had remained constant about him, and here he was ripping that away from me without any warning at all. I felt I had been tricked. I felt like I lost the only dad I knew. For weeks after I mourned the loss of my "real dad", and I don't think I ever really connected with this new clean-faced version of him. Because I was not prepared for the change, it stunned me, and left me feeling betrayed.

Autistics feel and function best when we have routine and predictability. We are particularly sensitive to unexpected changes of all kinds. Whether in or out of our control, unplanned events can trigger stress and anxiety. When the familiar pattern that we rely on for a sense of stability in a very chaotic and often overwhelming world is disrupted, many of us note feeling unable to regulate, accompanied by a deluge of panic. The consistency of our routines provides us with a sense of security and control that is otherwise out of our reach. As a result, unexpected or unplanned changes can lead to significant distress.

My dad and his haircut are just a mild instance of how distressing unplanned changes can be for Autistics. But I have survived many that weren't quite so easy for folks to dismiss. Death, for example, may be the ultimate, and most permanent, form of unexpected change. When death arrived in my life for the first time, I was totally unprepared.

I was 12 years old the year my Nana died. I had experienced some version of death and grief only once before, when our first cat, Lucifer, left us. As my relationship with animals is an intense one, how I processed that death was somehow more profound than what many might expect. For me, Lucifer was not just a pet; he was a confidant, a source of unconditional love and comfort in a world that often felt overwhelming and incomprehensible. His loss was not just the absence of a companion but a disruption in my entire world.

Nana was my dad's mother and my all-time favorite human, and we always had a ton of fun when we were together. She loved to cook for me and make my favorite of her specialties when I would come over. Scrambled eggs and onions, garlic mashed potatoes, chocolate pudding from scratch, and so many more. Nana and Pops lived really close to me and my mom, so I was there a lot! In fact, their apartment was the only other place I ever felt safe sleeping in. Mom would drop me off there in the morning on her way out, leaving me with a bag and a pickup time. And each time Nana would greet me like we hadn't seen each other in years, even though we never went more than two weeks without a visit.

Our days would be spent buying fun snacks and sneaking them into the movie theater or renting a movie for the VCR. Our preferred genre was horror, if not a good documentary, which can sometimes be the same thing. The gorier the better for us because we wanted to scare ourselves good. Then, magically,

Pops would arrive home exactly at dinner time, with fried chicken and potato salad for us from the deli in Manhattan where he was still the butcher despite having lost three fingers on one hand to the slicer many years back. Nana would set the table and we'd all sit down to eat together at their tiny kitchen table in Queens. When bedtime hit, Nana would kick Pops out of his bed and onto the den couch for the night and we would cozy up in their bed for more TV and some good sleep.

Nana was my very favorite person next to my mom and the only other person I could be myself with. At 12, I never stopped to picture my life without either of them, but as I would come to find out, death would come for Nana, and our sleepovers would end, and abruptly.

The day that my dad told me Nana was in the hospital wasn't memorable in any way. I was in my room at his house, and he came in and said that Nana was in the hospital and asked if I wanted to visit her. I had been in hospitals more than most as my dad was a hospital administrator and here's what I knew about hospitals: hospitals stink. Literally, the smell in a hospital is a special beast. It's some odd combo of cleaning product and sickness, except on the cafeteria floor, which smells a million times worse with its mix of hot food smells. Blech. But the sensory nightmares don't end with smell in hospitals. The beeps and announcements, along with so many people talking, crying, or yelling is an endless cacophony. And the lights? Well, I think "fluorescent" says everything you need to know.

Knowing Nana was sleeping in a bed in the middle of all that did not make me feel good, but at the same time, would it really help anything if I suffered through it, too? I decided she wouldn't want me to have to do that, and also, she wouldn't want me to see her all sick. After all, Nana was a beautiful, but vain, woman, who prided herself on her appearance, never setting foot outside without her full face of makeup done to perfection. I told my dad no thanks on that hospital visit and that I would visit her when she got home, without even the hint of an idea that she would never be home again.

I honestly don't remember how I found out that Nana had died. My brain probably decided it was too painful to hang onto. But I do remember the utter and complete confusion that I felt standing in the middle of family members at the cemetery, as shovel by shovel strangers piled dirt on the coffin.

Nobody had prepared me. Nobody had sat me down and explained that sometimes people go into the hospital and are too sick to come home, and that sometimes, they are so sick that they die. Asking me to visit Nana in the hospital without that bit of information had set me up for missing a last visit with my very favorite person, and I don't think that I have ever really recovered. I never got to tell her how much I loved her or how much I looked forward to our time together. I didn't get to hold her delicate hand one more time or take in her smell. I was just left with a giant void where she used to be and no further information. As I write this, I still have no idea what she was sick with or why she died.

To help Autistics manage unexpected changes, it's crucial to put strategies in place that can ease the transition through change and to reduce anxiety it can cause. This might include providing clear and early warnings of potential changes, the use of visual schedules, or the creation of social stories to explain new and unexpected situations, while doing your best to maintain as many elements as possible of the usual routine. Consistency in how we are taught to approach change, and transitions in general, can also be helpful. Don't forget that giving an Autistic time and space to safely process or offering objects of comfort during these times is also always appreciated.

Being Autistic in a world designed by and for the neuromajority can feel like being trapped on an out of control and utterly unpredictable rollercoaster. And not a sleek and fast cool rollercoaster, but one of those old rickety, squeaky wooden rollercoasters. Needless to say, Autistics don't have the privilege of feeling safe very often in the world. We are constantly looking out for ways to regulate ourselves by maintaining some control of our lives wherever we can. But that need for some amount of autonomy in our lives can quickly lead to unhealthy coping mechanisms surrounding one of the human requirements for survival: food.

The story of my father's unexpected transformation and the profound loss of my Nana illustrate the depth of impact that even seemingly minor changes can have on Autistics. These experiences aren't just about a haircut or a missed hospital visit; they're about the disruption of the familiar, the comfort, and the predictable.

Preparing your child for changes, big or small, is about providing a buffer against the unpredictability of the world, offering a sense of security in the midst of change. Clear communication, ample preparation, and a consistent routine can significantly alleviate the anxiety associated with change. It's about creating a safe space where your child can navigate the complexities of life with confidence and support.

As parents and caregivers, your role extends beyond guiding your child through the practicalities of life. It's about walking alongside them, understanding their unique needs and perspectives, and fostering a nurturing environment that celebrates their individuality. By doing so, you're not just helping your child cope with the world; you're empowering them to thrive in it, with all its unpredictability and change.

In the chapters to come, we will delve deeper into strategies and approaches that can help Autistics navigate life's changes more comfortably and we'll explore how to create a supportive environment that respects and honors the Autistic way of being— and there is no more Autistic way of being than a steaming hot serving of chicken nuggets and fries.

7
Chicken nuggets and fries

The perfection of McDonald's chicken nuggets is something to be marveled at, a savory symphony of taste and texture accompanied by instant comfort and joy. Each golden, crispy nugget is a bite of bliss, a delightful treasure, perfectly seasoned and cooked to tender, juicy excellence that pairs perfectly with the salty, savory goodness of their fries. The fries, with their ideal crunch on the outside and soft, fluffy insides, are the perfect companion to the magic of the nuggets. Dipping them both into a favorite sauce creates a harmony of flavors to delight your senses. For me, McDonald's chicken nuggets aren't just a meal, but a joyful escape that consistently brings meaningful pleasure and comfort to my life. And no matter how many times I go, eating nuggets and fries remains a cherished ritual that brings me guaranteed satisfaction with every bite. Whether it's a reward after a doctor's appointment or a quick treat to lift my spirits, McDonald's chicken nuggets remind me that simple pleasures can bring the greatest joy.

After decades of loyalty to McDonald's and their nuggets, I can finally say with confidence that I am not alone in my nugget worship. I have met no end to the number of Autistics who share my dedication. I don't have any data to support my guess, but I do believe I understand the Autistic appeal. McDonald's does consistency like no other. They get what we mean when we say we want it to be the same every time and they deliver it. McDonald's was the first to go all white meat, guaranteeing their internal sameness, and the timed fryer does the rest to create us the same darn nuggets we got the time before that, and the same darn nuggets we'll want again next time. A McDonald's nugget is a McDonald's nugget every single time at every single McDonald's. And if that's not the crux of a strong routine, I don't know what is.

My love of McDonald's started early. My mom learned early that I was particular about what I ate, but that if we found something I liked, she could serve it to me for every lunch or dinner every single day and I would happily sit down and eat it. I was not someone who liked variety, nor did I particularly feel inclined to try new foods as I am, by nature, a creature of habit who finds comfort only in routine. For most of my life under 12, I very happily ate three things: boxed cereal for breakfast, tuna sandwiches on white bread for lunch, and lightly breaded white meat chicken with tater tots for dinner.

The deviation from those items occurred on the occasions that my mom decided to "go out" and her mother would come over to babysit for the night. As these nights were a huge disruptor of my usual, I used to beg my mom not to go until we made the rule that if Grams was coming over to sit, she would take me to McDonald's for nuggets. With our negotiation complete, her nights out became more frequent and so did my trips with Grams to Mickey D's for comfort and solace.

Safe foods are a huge part of Autistic culture. They are something we openly discuss and claim with pride. Our safe foods, after all, make up the majority of the Autistic diet. There are no limits to what a safe food can be, but also no rules about how long a safe food will remain safe. Many of us experience some safe foods for life, while also having some safe foods that come and go with no rhyme or reason.

For Autistics, safe foods provide comfort, predictability, and sensory satisfaction in a world that often feels loud and overwhelming. Safe foods are more than just "preferred" meals; they are essential elements of daily living that offer us a much-needed sense of security, stability, and autonomy. Eating can be disruptive to us for any number of reasons. As eating is a multi-sensory activity, the texture, taste, color, smell, and even temperature of food can be critical to whether we can or cannot ingest a food. Our chosen safe foods, however, will typically have consistent qualities that align well with our sensory needs and tolerances and are predictable in their sensory input, which provides comfort while also reducing anxiety. Safe foods often become our only reliable source of nourishment as most other foods can trigger adverse sensory reactions or add to overwhelm by contributing to the chaos and discomfort of the world around us.

This is exactly what happened to me one Saturday morning at our local diner as I sat with a plate of eggs getting cold and hard on my plate. It was my dad's pick-up day, and our routine was to head to a local diner for breakfast as the first stop of our time together. I was pretty much allowed to order what I wanted, but I almost always ordered one scrambled egg and bacon with white toast. On this particular day I was really hungry and feeling kind of grown up, so I decided that I wanted to order two eggs and that I didn't want them scrambled, I wanted them like my dad got them, over. My dad hesitated. He is not a fan of wasted food and liked to remind me under his breath that my stomach was always "smaller than my mouth", whatever that was supposed to mean. But I insisted that I could indeed eat two eggs and that I was old enough to dip my toast even if I think egg yolks are gross. And with that I ordered. When our plates came, I was instantly overwhelmed by the size of the plate that two eggs came on. It looked like way more food than I imagined, and also, the eggs were sort of clear and goopy in some places. Not wanting to admit my dad was right, and also feeling a little embarrassed that I was feeling scared of the food on my plate. I could tell my mom those things but never my dad. So, I tried to eat, picking around the goopy eggs at the edges and eating all my toast and bacon, even the toast crusts and the raw fatty parts of the bacon. Hoping I had tackled enough to appease my dad, I stopped eating. But the eggs now sat on my plate virtually alone, like a glaring "Wasted Food" sign. My dad asked about my eggs, but before I could attempt an answer, his face turned red and full of rage. He had told me not to order this, but I did and now I had to eat it, all of it, he said. Over the course of the next ten minutes, I proceeded to try and get those eggs in my mouth and down my throat without much success. My final attempt sent me running to the restroom to vomit up my toast and bacon. When I came out, my face streaked with tears, my dad simply got up, paid the bill, and motioned me to the car, where we spent the rest of our drive to his apartment in shared, repentant silence.

The importance of respecting and understanding the concept of safe foods for Autistic individuals cannot be overstated. These foods are not just about picky eating; they are deeply intertwined with our individual sensory processing and our emotional well-being. Forcing or pressuring someone with autism to eat foods outside their comfort zone can lead to trauma via stress, anxiety, and even physical discomfort. Family members and other caregivers should acknowledge the validity of safe foods and strive to accommodate these preferences in various settings, rather than forcing us to "try new things" or "starving" us from our safe foods to make us eat something different. Additionally, forcing us to finish our plates or to eat even when we are not hungry can contribute to further struggles with food. These battles can, over time, lead to more serious conditions like eating disorders such as anorexia or avoidant/restrictive food intake disorder (ARFID). The unnecessary pressure and negative attention that too often surrounds Autistic eating habits has led to a stigma and stereotype around our love of "beige" palate that makes us self-conscience adults who may seek to eat in isolation rather than enjoying the pleasures of a meal with others.

After decades trying to defend and understand my personal eating do's and don'ts and lots of trial and error, with new safe foods making their way in and many old ones that I had to grieve the loss of. But my consistent go-to has and always will be some form of chicken nuggets and fries. Whenever I find myself having to eat somewhere when I am feeling otherwise overwhelmed or insecure, my go-to menu item will always be some form of fried white meat chicken and a friendly potato dish on the side.

A few years after my adult diagnosis, this would become a test of unmasking.

I went on my first official date at the age of almost 40. Up until then, I dated plenty of people that I hung out with but had never actually been out on a proper date. When I was finally asked, I still had all those weird first date conundrums. I worried about what to wear. I considered safety plans like any real New Yorker. And ultimately, I started to concern myself about what I should order. Garlic and pasta sauce are easy no-go's, but what about chicken tenders? Can an adult order chicken tenders on a first date? Maybe I should be sophisticated and order something that requires a knife and fork? Or maybe I should be a real lady and order a salad? I had no idea what the right thing was to do.

When the evening arrived, I parked my car still unsure what the right menu item might be. And as I walked to the pub door, I would get no more time to think about it because my date was on time and ready to greet me. We went inside and were seated with our menus. The time had come. In a huge leap of faith and a giant attempt to embrace my authenticity, I took a deep breath and ordered those tenders. I really liked this guy and I wanted to be able to enjoy our conversation without having to force myself to be something I am not, like fancy or ladylike. And, perhaps most importantly, I wanted this guy to like me for exactly who I am, not some imitation of who I think I should be. And that's what ordering my safe food really meant in that moment. Those tenders were my little rebellion against dating norms and my first attempt to be my authentic self in pursuit of connection.

Our evening was a ton of fun, and my date didn't even bat an eye about what I ordered. We laughed a lot and made plans for another night together the next week. When I got back in my car, I felt confident in myself, a little giddy, and full! All these years later, I can tell you for sure that what I ordered that night is not what my now husband remembers about our first date. Instead, he remembers how we laughed over the beer menu, never once talked about jobs, or had any awkward silences.

Understanding and support play a key role in ensuring that an Autistic feels respected and comfortable in their dietary choices, even if they are choosing safe foods. The goal should be fostering a positive relationship with food and enjoying eating experiences. Autistic people use safe foods to minimize chaos and create safety in the areas within their control. Regularly being forced to choose our comfort over being able to meet societal expectations. Recognizing and honoring Autistic safe foods helps us learn to regulate ourselves, but eating is just one of many complex sensory needs and wants that Autistics must learn to embrace.

Autistic safe foods illustrate a fundamental aspect of Autistic life: the deep connection to certain foods that provide not just nourishment, but a sense of safety, predictability, and comfort. For parents and caregivers, understanding and respecting this connection is crucial. It's not just about accommodating a preference; it's about acknowledging a sensory and emotional need that is as vital as any other aspect of care. It's a gesture that goes beyond the dinner table; it's a message of acceptance and understanding.

As we move into the next chapter, we'll delve deeper into the various sensory experiences and needs that define the Autistic experience. From the textures of fabrics to the intensity of sounds, each aspect plays a crucial role in shaping the daily lives of Autistic individuals. By understanding these sensory intricacies, we can create more accommodating and supportive environments, where Autistic individuals can thrive and find joy in their unique way of interacting with the world.

8
Sensory hellscapes

Showering is my arch nemesis. We have been in a heated battle since I graduated from baths, and most of the time when we face off, I end up slinking away damp and defeated. Showering has lots of supporters. From parents arming their kids against never-ending germs to beautiful women looking to smell like they stepped out of a florist, showering need not look far to find fans. But for me, showering offers very little to be desired. Because, along with the overwhelming call on my executive functioning, showering brings with it a complex sensory nightmare every single time.

Imagine that you are on your couch reading or scrolling through your phone in your comfy home clothes and the time for a shower arrives. You get up off the couch and head to the bathroom with its bright lights and cold floors. With your first breath in, a cacophony of smells hits your nose. The light floral notes of soap mingle with the minty freshness of toothpaste, vaguely covering the scent of bleach from the last cleaning day. You begin to undress. Each cozy, well-worn item on your person must be removed and tossed to the floor, exposing you to the cool air and leaving you vulnerable. You reach into the shower, used not too long ago by a household member, to turn on the water, and as you do so, the cold beads of water left on the curtain liner drag along your uncovered arm, chilling you to your core. After methodically testing the water temperature, you carefully step into the shower, and despite all of your efforts, your skin is never quite prepared for the shock of the water hitting you all over and all at once. Now begins the onslaught of products, each smelling just a little chemically fresh even though they claim to be "unscented". Throughout your shower, those smells layer and intensify as they comingle in the thick humid air surrounding you now. Breathing is unpleasant.

Shampoo, conditioner, body wash, face wash…did you remember to wash everything in the correct order? Fairly sure you have done all you can do, it's time to turn off the water that you have adjusted to, and once again face what feels like even colder air. As you step out, the shower curtain liner drags along your lower leg like it is trying to keep you there just a little longer. Once free, the drying begins. Your wet hair is leaving water trails down your back, so you quickly wrap it up in a towel. Next, you take a second towel and carefully dry all the parts of yourself that you just scrubbed clean. Out of breath and exhausted, be it clean and dry, you put on your deodorant, brush your hair, moisturize, or whatever your post-shower product routine may be. Then, finally, with your last bit of energy, you throw on a robe or get dressed for the day, knowing that tomorrow you are expected to do it all over again.

Saying that I hate showering is not only an understatement but also something about me that gets misunderstood a lot. When folks know that I am an Autistic that hates to shower they immediately assume that I like being dirty and must walk around leaving visible fingerprints, and stinking up rooms, with a giant dirt storm following me, kind of like Pig-Pen from a Charlie Brown cartoon. In reality, I am, and always have been, a very neat, clean, and hygienically aware human. Meaning, just because I hate showering, doesn't mean that I don't do it. I hate eating most of the time, too, but I have yet to starve myself to death. I have always showered every single day with military precision until I realized just a few years ago that if I wasn't out digging ditches for a living, I could skip a shower every once in a while. Now I allow myself the privilege of skipping the shower nightmare on days when I am otherwise overloaded or just too exhausted to make it through a shower without triggering a meltdown.

When faced with a shower day, I feel immediate dread. First, because I know the inevitable sensory explosion ahead, and second because I know that it will automatically deplete my energy, leaving me with a much more limited supply for whatever else I might try to accomplish that day. Similarly, if I attempt to shower on a day that I am otherwise overextended, it becomes a near-impossible task, and on those days, I have learned to treat myself with kindness and let the shower wait for the next day.

As I kid, I could never express this clearly. Instead, I would say things like, "I don't want to shower", or "Not now", when what I was trying to say was, "Showering is too much" and "I am too tired."Though often met with a sigh, our family battles over bathing were never our worst, but for a lot of Autistic families the battles that happen over hygiene are a constant and ongoing war of miscommunication. Not having the language to express the sensory intensity of the demands of bathing, many of us protest, refuse showering altogether, or shower under duress, building up discomfort, resentment, dread, and sometimes even phobias.

This is a classic misunderstanding, with the Autistic person trying to communicate how intense the experience is and the parent just wanting their kid to get clean and not understanding what is so awful about the process.

On days when the adult world would demand a shower before other draining activities like family events or the almighty errands, I could feel my heart crumble, knowing that a shower on top of all those other things would simply be "too much". Moreover, it felt like an unnecessary burden placed on top of an already large demand for my energy. How could I be expected to regulate that?

The short answer is, I couldn't. Many of my regular meltdowns had their origin in the shower, but they came to full maturity with the epic challenge posed by getting dressed, especially when I had to dress "appropriately" for some socially heavy adult-oriented event, like the wedding I had to attend at six years old for some family member I saw at most twice a year. While I don't remember exactly whose wedding it was that we had to attend, I do remember the outfit that I wore with perfect detail. It was a black long-sleeved top with gold roses on the front and a little petal skirt to match. The entire outfit was made out of sweatshirt material, and I absolutely loved it. It was the first time that I liked my clothes and felt comfortable in them. The problem with the outfit was that I was also "supposed to" wear tights and shoes with it and I didn't do shoes and socks. My mom had gone to so many stores and I had tried on so many outfits for this event, and finally we were able to agree on this one. However, in all the times I had tried it on, she had never once mentioned these tights and shoes requirements.

The day of the event arrived, and it began with an early morning shower, never a sign that goodness lies ahead. After said shower it was on to a small breakfast of pop tarts, cold, and then getting dressed. I was excited to finally be allowed to wear sweats to a fancy event and got dressed in a flash, skipping through the house with ease. As Mom went to put on my coat, she looked down and realized I had nothing on my legs and feet. She had left out my thick black wool tights and my shiny, stiff patent leather Mary Jane shoes, and I had just left them there. Why would I ruin a perfectly good outfit by suffocating my legs with tights and squishing my toes inside shoes? My toes need to wiggle, and my legs need freedom to bend, I protested. But my mom insisted that tights and shoes were a must. I was already overloaded by my earlier shower and now uncomfortable, unplanned expectations were suddenly being placed on me. Try as might I could not get the tights on without tears, and before I could even try for a shoe, I was in full meltdown.

I know we went to the wedding, and I know I wore the outfit with the tights and shoes, because my pouty, red-faced self is in all the photos, my misery captured for posterity. I also know that as soon as those photos were taken, I ran to the bathroom and ripped up those tights, tossing them in the trash with relief. Then, barefoot, I ran to our assigned table and threw my shoes under it, hoping they would get left behind when we finally made our way home.

With sensory sensitivities like mine, the decision about when I shower and what I wear has a huge impact. It can make the difference between accomplishing my goals and not being able to meet them. To regulate both my energy and my sensory input,

I have to make sure to prioritize my comfort level over everything else. Choosing comfort and regulation over societal expectations is empowering for Autistic individuals as all too often social norms and expectations can be overwhelming, demanding conformity in ways that are unnatural or uncomfortable for us. When we don't have the freedom to choose comfort, it often negatively impacts everything, and everyone, we encounter. It's physically and emotionally painful and comes at great cost to our wellbeing. While, for the adults in charge, giving us the autonomy to make comfort a priority comes at virtually no physical, financial, or social cost.

One of the ways I learned to get around the seemingly innumerable and unattainable social expectations around dressing "appropriately" was to create uniforms for myself. I created uniforms by finding socially acceptable clothes that were also comfortable and wearing the same thing in different versions, every single day. Much like with food, this became a reliable way to get dressed that took little energy to execute. As a kid, that would mean owning the same t-shirt in many different colors and a few pairs of overalls or leggings to go with them. My high school uniform was jeans from the thrift store, an all-cotton black t-shirt with a flannel over it, and my Doc Martin six-hole boots, and remained as such until well into my 30s. Uniforms work for Autistics, because they always feel and fit the same, but there is more to it than just that.

I have always been drawn to the color black. It exudes safety and comfort to me and has long been my clothing color of choice. Bright colors make me feel physically ill to wear, right along with unnatural fabrics. Yet I love bright colors for my hair, which

I started dying crazy colors at the age of 12. For me, what I choose to wear and how I look on the outside is my greatest rebellion while also being my longest form of silent self-expression.

This can be confusing for adults. "Why", they think, "would she refuse to wear that lovely lime green shirt I bought her last week, and then this week want to dye her hair that exact color?" To parents, teachers, and caregivers, these can seem like confusing contradictions. How is it that I could wear sturdy Doc Martins but I couldn't stand the feeling of those Mary Janes? Why did I hate colorful clothes but insist on it in my hair? I wasn't being defiant or difficult, I was managing my energy.

Autistics, I often explain in my corporate trainings, are extremely energy efficient. For me, the Doc Martins were part of my identity. I liked people who wore Docs. I liked the brand and what it stood for. I liked how I felt when I looked at my feet in them. Wearing Docs gave me a little bit of energy and took almost none away. Those Mary Janes on the other hand were not "me". They weren't how I saw myself or how I wanted to be seen. The style felt like the opposite of me. And the unconscious effect of this was that I would notice all the places the hard leather cut into my sensitive skin (even through those awful tights!). The Mary Janes zapped me of energy, and the lower my energy got the less I could tolerate the negative sensory input. To a non-Autistic outsider, the discrepancies might not make sense, but inside the Autistic body, I can assure you, there is no denying it.

From the overwhelming experience of showering to the complexities of choosing clothing, these sensory challenges are not mere inconveniences but significant hurdles in daily life. The coping mechanisms developed, like creating personal uniforms or adjusting hygiene routines, are not just about comfort, but essential strategies for managing sensory overload and maintaining energy levels.

For Autistics, embracing personal comfort means acknowledging and respecting our unique sensory needs, as well as our differing communication styles and relationship preferences. It involves the courageous act of prioritizing one's mental and emotional well-being over the pressure to fit into a conventional mold. This approach not only fosters self-acceptance but also challenges societal norms, promoting a more inclusive and understanding environment. By choosing our own comfort above all else, Autistics can thrive in our authenticity, making for a more fulfilling and less stressful life.

For parents, understanding the sensory world of your Autistic child is crucial. Showering, dressing, and other daily activities can be overwhelming due to sensory issues, and your child's responses are not acts of defiance but ways of coping. Recognizing and respecting these sensitivities, and adapting routines to reduce sensory overload, can greatly aid your child's comfort and ability to function.

This exploration into sensory sensitivities sets the stage for the next chapter, which delves into the concept of masking. Masking is the act of concealing one's Autistic traits to blend into neurotypical society. Understanding sensory sensitivities is crucial in comprehending why masking is a common practice among Autistics.

Of course, now I know what was going on for me all those years ago when it came to bathing and dressing. They were both areas where the outside demand was greater than any benefit I was receiving. Over time, I was teaching myself to ignore my needs in an effort to please the outside world. In essence, I was intentionally making myself uncomfortable for the comfort of those around me. Suffering, while the adults in my life judged whether what I looked like was acceptable to them. All of my refusing to get dressed or take a shower was simply my best attempt to verbalize my needs and not because I liked being stubborn, difficult, or dirty. I was constantly in search of sensory relief and energy regulation, and ignoring my unmet needs so regularly meant that my dysregulation would show itself in other parts of my life, as well.

9
The price of pretending

"Tsk, tsk, tsk, tsk…" Just inside every classroom of P.S. 221, hanging above the door, sat the same giant General Electric wall clock. Each one with its identical brown round metal frame, stalwart and severe black Arabic numbers, the slow-moving pointy black hands, and the powder-blue second hand that worked its way around the face with its regular judgmental tsk sound marking the expected cadence of each room. Convinced they were built to move more slowly, I hated those clocks and spent most of each day not only trying to ignore the second hand that nobody else seemed to hear, but also desperately trying to move time with the power of my stare like Dr Jean Grey from the X-Men. But try as I might, the big hands never responded to my telekinetic efforts encouraging them forward, and the second hand continued to judge its way methodically through the day no matter how hard I tried to will it silent.

My only escape was a trip to the bathroom, which I did with a regularity that would make that annoying second hand proud. The only obstacle to my regular lavatory respite sessions was "The Pass". It was the policy in my school that any student in the hallway during class had to have "The Pass" from the teacher on their person. Each classroom had its own version of "The Pass" designed by the teacher and only one person could have possession of "The Pass" at any given moment. "The Pass" was as revered as the hidden immunity idols on the TV show "Survivor" and functioned similarly. You had to earn the right to possess "The Pass" and you did your best to hold onto it for as long as possible as it provided temporary immunity in a game you didn't stand a chance at winning.

Yet, despite how coveted "The Pass" was, and even though it would mean battling situational mutism to ask for it, the peace and privacy offered by a darkened bathroom stall and the regulation provided by the short walk back and forth were enough incentive to raise my hand multiple times a day. So often in fact, that as one teacher handed me "The Pass", she said, "You can't possibly need to go to the bathroom again." Taking "The Pass" from the corner of her desk, I quietly mumbled "You can't possibly know that", and off I went to sit silently in a stall yet again.

With hindsight, it's clear to see that I was in desperate need of regular breaks in my day to regulate. It's also clear to see that I didn't feel like my teachers would understand that at all. Rather than feeling secure that the adults around me would support me, I learned to lie about, hide, and mask my needs. The clear message around this was that my needs were nowhere near as important as doing what I was supposed to do like everyone else was doing and being a "good girl". Over time, this cycle became so ingrained that it evolved into my brain no longer receiving my own body signals in time or at all, while also simultaneously teaching me to ignore my natural instincts that may have remained. Learning to mask my needs at such an early age quite literally destroyed my eighth sense, interoception.

Interoception is the internal sensory system that allows the brain to perceive and understand physical sensations arising within our own bodies (Garfinkel et al., 2016). This includes the ability to recognize and interpret a wide range of internal signals such as hunger, thirst, heart rate, and temperature. Unlike other senses like sight and hearing, interoception focuses on the body's internal state, which means it plays a crucial role in maintaining regulation and emotional well-being. Interoception is also closely linked with our emotional experience and self-awareness, as the interpretation of these internal signals can influence our response time and decision-making abilities. For example, the sensation of a racing heart might be interpreted as anxiety or excitement, depending on the context and individual awareness.

Interoception has a significant connection to autism. Not surprisingly, many Autistics report that they experience interoception differently. These differences can look like difficulty recognizing or interpreting internal bodily sensations, like pain, hunger, or changes in heart rate. This can then impact if and how we are able to meet our physical needs. Since interoception is closely linked to emotional awareness and regulation, difficulties in interoceptive processing can also affect the emotional experience of Autistics. We can struggle with alexithymia, which is when we have challenges naming our emotions, and we can also struggle understanding the why behind our feelings, both of which can lead to further struggles with emotional regulation. That's probably the reason why I wanted to go to the bathroom so often, to hide from the classroom clock and other overstimulating sounds and sights. While I wasn't able to identify or articulate what was causing me discomfort, or even really recognize that I was uncomfortable, something didn't feel right, and I had the urge to get away.

In the quiet of the bathroom, everything would slow down. My body would decompress, and I was able to take in large breaths that always ended in an audible sigh of relief. Alone in the stall, I felt comfortable, which tells me now just how uncomfortable I was the rest of my day. Knowing my time was limited outside the classroom, those moments of stall silence were the only way I was able to regulate throughout the day. The rest of the time I would spend in a state of dysregulation that would build up and up and up until the General Electric clock hit 3 pm. This meant the majority of my school-day energy was spent actively learning to ignore my needs.

Since the interoceptive system guides many of our subconscious decisions, having challenges in this area can lead to difficulties in self-regulation and decision-making. It's not just about recognizing when to eat or sleep, but also about understanding and responding to emotional states. This variation in interoceptive awareness can impact daily life in numerous ways. This can lead to misunderstandings and feelings of isolation. Cultivating interoceptive awareness can help us understand our unique sensory processing experiences and can greatly improve our overall quality of life without having to hide behind tricks like trips to the bathroom.

Beyond those bathroom breaks, there were many other scenarios I had to learn to mask through at a very young age. Eye contact is a big one for the neuromajority. More than any other part of communicating, the importance of maintaining eye contact during conversation is something that I will simply never understand. To this day, I just do not get what staring into another person's eyeballs has to do with how engaged you are in the conversation at hand. But over time I learned that eye contact is essential in order for non-Autistics to feel you are paying attention to them. And so, like many of us, I learned to mimic eye contact for the comfort of the neuromajority.

Eye contact is painful for me. It literally makes my insides contract and my brain scream. Animals seem to experience eye contact the way Autistics do, as a threat, not something you do in hopes of keeping others around. In the early years, it was just too painful to answer the demands of "look at me when I am talking", so I would just repeat back the last sentence spoken to express that I had indeed been listening. But the older I got, the fiercer the demands for eye contact got and the expectation that eye contact was required for speaking as well as listening was added. It was around this time that I discovered that if I just concentrated on the space between people's eyebrows during conversations, I was mimicking eye contact close enough to actually pass for doing it.

The lesson I was being taught was to tone down my Autisticness for everyone else's comfort. My comfort was less important. I learned from adults that things like spinning, repeating phrases out loud, and flapping my hands were not really "approved" behaviors if you are looking to minimize your differences. I forced myself to replace those natural means of regulation with smaller gestures like finger tapping or making fists in my pockets, and invisible stims like biting the inside of my mouth and lips and wiggling my toes in my shoes. All day long I would keep it small and hold it in, until I was home where it was safe to be me. Quiet at school all day long, I worked so hard to be a "good girl" that by the time I got home I was ready to explode and desperate for joy.

In order to fit in, I spent most of my lifetime suppressing my authentic self and trying on personas like costumes to feel like I belonged somewhere. It was like I was a duck living with a family of swans and I was doing whatever I could to look and act like all the other swans. This little "dress up and pretend to not be myself" routine is now known more commonly as masking.

Masking, or "social camouflaging", is a coping mechanism where Autistics consciously or unconsciously conceal or modify their Autistic traits in an effort to conform to societal expectations and/ or to fit in with their peers. Many Autistic females become highly skilled, partly due to social pressures earlier on in development and the different ways that autism is interpreted in males and females (Parish-Morris et al., 2017). Masking can manifest in a variety of ways, such as mimicking neuro-normative social behavior, hiding or minimizing Autistic traits, scripting or rehearsing social narratives, suppressing needs and emotions, forcing eye contact, and adapting personas to fit in with particular social groups or based on the people we are with.

Masking has significant mental health implications and is the leading cause of burnout for Autistic adults (South, Costa, & McMorris, 2021). While masking is often a way to navigate social situations more easily, it often leads to increased stress, anxiety, and exhaustion. Long-term masking contributes to a loss of personal identity and an overall lack of self-esteem, and for many is the cause of delayed identification of autism, especially in females. Masking is an unsustainable response to trauma that over a long period of time can lead to an inability to know who you are and what you need without it. Lost, we often find ourselves doing things that do not align with who we really are in an effort to find belonging.

By the time I reached high school, I was a well-practiced masker. So good, that I often wondered if I still existed or if the persona that I was wearing so much of the time was actually me. It was the early 1990s and my uniform of choice was modeled directly after Eddie Vedder's closet. Pearl Jam was, and still is, my favorite band and I loved how androgenous and purposefully messy the grunge vibe let me be. My flannels, tees, and Docs clearly expressed my approach to the world, there but not really thrilled about it. My uniform had other perks. It not only set me apart from the popular mean girls and the egocentric athletes, but it also stated that I understood my status as a weirdo, which meant other weirdos knew I was one of them.

With my high school persona cemented as the rebellious outcast, I had finally begun to experience belonging for the first time, and it was magical. For the first time in my life, I had a group of friends that liked me for my weirdness, and I felt like

I was home. Never wanting to risk this miraculous arrangement, it became my sole mission to make sure that I kept my place in our friend group. We proudly moped the halls together, only looking up from the floor to open our lockers. We met in odd corners of school to congregate, cut class, and smoke cigarettes. We met in each other's basements to smoke joints and drink, and we spent hours in one car or another just driving around listening to music.

While cutting class was something I could get behind, some of the other things that went along with my new persona weren't necessarily aligned with who I was on the inside. Smoking was gross and made me feel sick. The smell of it on my clothes made me queasy, and paying someone to buy them for me made me anxious. But everyone in our group smoked and, therefore, so did I, all the while telling myself I liked it. It was the same with beer and alcohol. I didn't like the taste and I didn't really like the hot, dizzy way it made me feel. But that's what we did on weekends, figure out how to get alcohol, agree on where to meet to drink it, and then do that, and so I did. And by the time high school was coming to an end, I had stopped caring about the learning part, absorbed that I was a broken weirdo, and believed that I would never go to college. But none of that bothered me; I just wanted to feel like I belonged.

I'm sure this was a rough time for both of my parents. I am a rule follower by nature, so I think they were taken by surprise by how easily I was able to break them when it came to my friends. They had the typical rebellious teen on their hands and had all the strife that comes with it. But they were missing one giant piece of the pie: the why behind my rebellion. Neither of them knew that autism was on board, so to them I was doing all of this for attention or to be difficult. I was just a bad kid. But what they didn't understand was that I desperately needed to experience connection with my peers and that just making sure I was invited to places was enough to keep me as your friend. I had no understanding of who I was outside of the rebellion and no love for who I was underneath my outcast mask.

The importance of experiencing true belonging and having safe spaces to be one's authentic self cannot be overstated, especially for those who routinely feel the need to engage in masking, like Autistics. The act of concealing, minimizing, or changing yourself to conform to societal norms and expectations that do not come naturally to you demands immense effort and energy. It involves constant monitoring and adjusting your actions, speech, body language, facial expressions, and more, which can be both mentally and emotionally draining. This continuous effort can lead to increased stress, anxiety, and an overarching sense of isolation. In contrast, having a safe space where one can be unapologetically authentic allows for a significant reduction in this mental burden.

The primary assignment for parents and caregivers of Autistic people is to create spaces where we are free to be ourselves. By creating a space where Autistics can express themselves freely and be exactly who they are without fear of judgment, you can not only alleviate the stress associated with masking but also contribute profoundly to their self-esteem and identity development. It fosters a sense of belonging and acceptance, crucial for mental and emotional well-being. Acceptance at home is the foundation for security and confidence that enables us to explore and engage who we really are inside. Without the freedom and security of safe spaces to be ourselves, we are left to experience only the negative consequences of unmasking in front of others.

10
Brightness and burnout

For decades, I was denied my own reality. To me, bright light is painful and for most of my life the adults around me told me that that wasn't possible. Invalidated, whenever I found myself faced with a brightly lit room or outside in the direct sunlight for long periods, I would prepare myself to be plagued with monster head pain for hours afterwards. The kind of head pain that stops you from all other activity and forces you to lay down in whatever dark corner is closest. A pain so demanding that it makes you hot and queasy while forcing you to focus on only one task, breathing.

"Migraines", the doctor said to me and mom. My mom quickly clarified, "In a nine-year-old?", she asked. The doctor nodded in confirmation as he went on to explain that it's rare for children but could be an early sign of a brain tumor, so he ordered me my very first MRI. He said it to us like he was buying me a present, but MRI, or magnetic resonance imaging, is anything but a gift for an undiagnosed Autistic.

I had that first MRI at the hospital that my dad worked at, so both parents were with me, and it was weird. Seeing them together made me uncomfortable, like my two worlds colliding, even though they had spent years as a couple before I came into exist-ence. Still, it was out of routine and unsettling. Little did I know that in mere moments I would be begging for them both to make it stop.

We were down in the basement for this event, as that is where they housed the then giant metal tube that was an MRI machine in the 1980s. You can take a moment to Google image search the beast of which I speak. It was a behemoth monster of a machine with a tube-like opening in the front and it took up most of the room we were in. They had me put on a gown on arrival and I had kept on my socks because the floor was cold linoleum tile. A medical person of some kind helped me up into the machine and had me lay flat. He strapped my head down into a mask that kept my head and neck still. Next, he strapped down my wrists and ankles to keep my nine-year-old body from wiggling. Even though I couldn't look up, I knew both my parents were watching through the window I had seen on my way into the room. The medical person said he was going to leave the room, but that he would talk to me through a microphone from the other side of the window, and that he would be able to hear me. He told me that if I got nervous, I could look up using just my eyes and there was a mirror on my mask that was pointed so that I could see just my feet. I tried it out and it seemed to work.

With that, he said we would begin and the table I was strapped to started to slowly slide into the tube opening. Behind my head I heard the giant machine rumble to life. With a final bump, I had slid entirely into the tube. I tried the mirror and could barely make out my feet and the opening to freedom. Then came the bang-ing. It surrounded me and there was no escape. And aggressive knocking was added to the banging and the panic began to rise from my gut.

Without warning, I found myself screaming for my parents in sheer and utter terror. In moments, or hours, the table began to slide out and I found my father standing next to me holding my foot as they unstrapped me. I was then able to see my mom through the window. She was crying and mouthing I'm sorry.

I tried the MRI a few more times that day but could not complete it. And the headache it left me with was too awful for it to be ironic. Eventually I was sedated for the procedure, and it came back negative, meaning there was no visible tumor or cause for my head pain. Relieved it wasn't cancer, my parents started me on a protocol for migraines, which included lots of medications not really intended for growing brains. And on an annual basis, I would be traumatized and sedated for an MRI just to make sure that a tumor hadn't appeared.

Decades later, still believing that I suffered with near constant migraine headaches, medication and all, my autism diagnosis would enter the picture. With it I would learn about my sensory sensitivities and figure out my triggers, slowly creating a life that didn't make me feel like I was under attack from the world. As I got to know myself again, and made changes to reflect my needs, my headaches started to get less and less frequent. Soon, I was down to only one big headache a month triggered by menstruation and that was it.

After years of treating myself for migraines, it became clear that not all my headaches were migraines but were actually sensory-overload headaches. Moreover, understanding the source of my headaches validated decades of knowing that yes, for me, light is painful. Fortunately, when I learned how to regulate my sensory environment thanks to my autism diagnosis, those headaches all but disappeared.

Autism can have significant and often underappreciated impacts on physical health, extending beyond the more commonly discussed psychological and social challenges. For example, Autistic individuals frequently experience gastrointestinal issues, headaches, and insomnia. These physical manifestations may be linked to the heightened levels of stress and anxiety commonly experienced by Autistic individuals, as we face overwhelming social demands and sensory stimuli in the world around us. This chronic anxiety and stress can lead to elevated cortisol levels, a hormone associated with stress response, which in turn can contribute to the development of conditions like high blood pressure and cardiovascular issues.

Additionally, autism can co-occur with other conditions that may be overlooked, such as hypermobile Ehlers-Danlos Syndrome (hEDS), a connective tissue disorder. The overlap of symptoms between autism and such conditions can complicate diagnoses and treatment, leading to instances of medical gaslighting where patients' symptoms are dismissed or misdiagnosed. This lack of recognition and appropriate care for co-occurring conditions not only exacerbates physical health issues but can also contribute to a sense of isolation and misunderstanding for Autistics. With our realities invalidated yet again, many of us end up masking our physical discomfort and ignoring our needs completely.

My headaches and the doctor appointments that went with them often meant missing school. And while I loved a good excuse to miss a school day, returning afterwards was torture. Not only was all the sensory input that much louder after a day away, but I would have also missed important social information that I desperately needed to maintain my fitting-in mask. A day away for the doctor could mean that I missed a funny story or a teacher wearing a bad outfit or a fire drill where the fire department actually came. Any and all of those things plus many others would leave me out of the loop, behind on the inside jokes, and bring attention to the many differences I was working so hard to hide. As much as I hated school, missing school gave me unruly anxiety.

Each week, I was left to decide which was worse, going to school or the anxiety from the day off. As I got older and the social demands became more complex, one day out of school a week wasn't enough for my brain to regulate. By fifth and sixth grades, the headaches were coming so often that the only way I could get a break from them was to stay home at least two days in a row, one with the pain and the one without it to recharge and enjoy. And with twice as many days out, the social anxiety of the return doubled, too. What did I miss? Would the other girls ask why I was out? Would they judge me for the truth? Should I lie instead? Before long, two days out become three, then four, the social anxiety mounting with each day missed. Then when I did come back, I was the weird sick kid, so messed up she missed too much school. So broken she can't fit in or keep up. With that, five days out became two weeks and then a month, and then even my mom wasn't happy with me. Furious, she explained to me about truant officers and her getting in trouble with the police. But I couldn't imagine going back. There would be so many stares, so many questions, and so much EVERYTHING.

I spent most of seventh and eighth grades classified as a school refuser, a behavioral problem child. The truant officer and the police did eventually come to my house, but it wasn't enough to scare me back out into the world. They sent me a homeschool teacher four days a week for six hours a day. I watched TV while she sat in my dining room, doing only the homework that I liked. They sent me to three different alternative schools, all of which I refused to attend after one or two days. Everything was just too much, and I was just too tired.

It took me years after my autism diagnosis to understand that the year and a half that I was a "school refuser" was in reality my first experience with Autistic burnout. Autistic burnout is a significant, debilitating, total exhaustion experienced by Autistic individuals. It differs from ordinary burnout in its causes, symptoms, and what it takes to heal from it. It is recognized by lengthy and intense mental, physical, and emotional exhaustion, which is usually accompanied by a loss of or reduction in skills and abilities.

Though the causes of Autistic burnout are complex, it is most often rooted in the cumulative effect of the constant effort required to navigate a world designed for the neuromajority. This includes the pressure of social interactions, the effort required to mask Autistic traits to fit into societal expectations, and the sensory overload that can come from everyday environments. Unlike ordinary burnout, which is often related to workplace stress, Autistic burnout is often the direct result of prolonged and sustained masking, social demands, and exposure to uncontrolled sensory inputs without the ability to regulate.

Symptoms of Autistic burnout can include, but are not limited to, chronic fatigue, reduced tolerance for stimuli, increased irritability, depression, anxiety, and a noticeable decline in skills and abilities. It's important to note that these symptoms are often misinterpreted as a "regression" in skills, instead of the response to prolonged stress that it is. The impact of Autistic burnout can be profound, as it affects an individual's ability to function in almost all aspects of life, including work, school, and personal relationships.

Recovery from Autistic burnout requires a personalized approach, acknowledging the unique needs and experiences of the individual. This may involve reducing demands, implementing coping strategies for sensory sensitivities, and providing support in daily activities. Recovery can also be a lengthy process. It can take years to find yourself in burnout, and likewise, it can take years to get better, but recovery is impossible without understanding and support from family, friends, and trusted professionals.

Validating physical discomfort and sensory overload is crucial, especially for individuals with a hyper-connected, Autistic brain. Though neither of my parents experienced sensory sensitivities, when I shared with them that light was a source of pain for me, I would have loved a different response from them. For instance, knowing light is a source of pain or discomfort for me, it would have been really helpful for them to teach me how to proactively manage my sensitivity by carrying sunglasses as a regulatory tool everywhere. If they had embedded in my brain that I should always bring my sunglasses, instead of invalidating my reality, I would have been spared a good number of those "migraines" that I was having from sensory overload.

Unlike the brains of the neuromajority, Autistic brains often process a large amount of information without filtering it at all. While this can lead to painful sensory overload, it can also lead to intensely pleasurable sensory experiences. By not masking our sensory experiences and instead employing healthy regulation strategies, Autistics can learn to not only prevent burnout but also discover unimaginable sources of sensory joy. These strategies might include the use of headphones with or without music, designated quiet times, or engaging in activities that soothe and satisfy our unique sensory needs. Embracing our sensory sensitivities allows us more authentic interaction with the world around us. By respecting the Autistic brain's innate sensory processing, the challenge it can represent easily transforms into an opportunity for self-discovery and experimentation with activities that do help us to regulate, like the ones in the next chapter.

11
Discovering regulation

Our local public park was located directly next to the school district's regional special education school. Growing up, my "normal" friends and I would watch the kids who attended as they were wheeled or walked holding hands with an aid to the "short buses" that NYC used for wheelchair accessibility at the end of their school day. Back in the 1980s it was the practice to keep Disabled children in their own schools and not just in their own classrooms. Distance from difference was a priority back then. When my friends and I would get occasional glimpses of the "special needs" kids, we were fascinated and could not help but watch.

I was drawn to watching the few Deaf kids in the group of children when we saw them. I was fascinated by the ease with which they communicated without ever making a sound. That, silently, they could share jokes or worries or knowing glances. Their secret language of sign was so graceful to watch and so very fast but fluid. They would laugh together at jokes nobody heard and they would share looks of knowing together that I had never experienced. For years I watched with jealousy of their silent world, wishing mine was just half as quiet while also envying how easily they seemed to control their hands, while my hands seemed to have minds of their own. Sign language was beautiful to watch, and I longed for a way to communicate that felt more natural to me than speech. But more than anything else, I was jealous of their private world and their shared language that brought them closer together while keeping the rest of the world out. I was as envious of their belonging as I was of the quiet world that they got to live in.

I often found myself experimenting with blocking out sounds. I'd stick my fingers in my ears or stuff cotton balls into my ears for hours. And I would mimic sign language as an additional stim. I loved how muted the world became when I blocked out sounds. My brain would be still, finding regulation in the lack of auditory input while keeping my hands moving as an additional relief. Blocking out sounds was my first innocent attempt to self-regulate, in a way that actually worked for me and at a time well before Bose released their trendy noise-canceling headphones. But it was something I could not rely on outside of the house.

The first publicly acceptable way I learned to self-regulate was by swimming. Being underwater mimicked my earlier efforts to block out sounds but was even better. Moving my whole body was much more regulating than just moving my hands and there is nothing quieter and more peaceful than being fully underwater. My body and brain relished the weightlessness that full submersion in water brings. It simultaneously shuts out the whole world while forcing you to keep moving to stay alive. Swimming, in its most basic form, was my preferred stim for years. I spent as much time in the water as I could, loving summer only for its regular pool access.

I spent endless hours in the pool alone, and I liked it that way. As an only child, it was my favorite privilege that I got to play alone because it gave me much-needed time for recovery and recharge without the anxiety of pleasing others. I loved my solo pool time and still do. I could lose myself in my own world, let my imagination have at it, and there were nobody else's needs to consider. I had developed the habit of imagining I was in a movie in my head, though I was always the narrator of the imaginary storyline and never the main character. Being already a consummate observer, and naturally skilled at pattern recognition, it was comfortable for me to "play characters" in these underwater "films", trying on the body language and facial expressions of people I had seen, away from the judging eyes of both adults and my peers. Those hours alone in the pool were critical periods of recharge and alone time that I desperately needed, and swimming was the perfect, adult-approved activity to explore my inner world without interruption.

Autistics often have unique motivations and preferences regarding our free time and our need for solitude to recharge and regulate. This divergence from the neuromajority is not rooted in narcissism, but rather in our profound need for self-regulation in a very loud world. Many Autistic individuals will gravitate towards activities and stims that provide sensory comfort, or cognitive engagement, or both, which may appear unconventional or overly focused to others. Our choices are often sparked by a deep-seated need to balance our internal sensory and emotional states. The pursuit of these activities is often less about self-indulgence and more about seeking a sense of balance that can be elusive in a world not tailored to our Autistic sensibilities.

When an Autistic individual finds a self-regulatory stimming behavior (a repetitive body movement or noise) that is both fulfilling and socially acceptable, they might engage in it with abundance. Much like an alcoholic at an open bar, when we find a stim that checks those two boxes, excess is on the menu. However, the key distinction lies in our underlying motivation. Autistic individuals are not acting out of a desire to be self-centered or manipulative; our actions are motivated by a desperate search for sensory and emotional regulation. Discovering a stim that provides relief and fits within social norms can be rare, and when it happens, the desire to maintain that state of comfort can be overwhelming. This relentless pursuit of regulatory activities is not a choice, but a necessary response to the complex challenges faced in navigating a world that often feels overwhelming and unpredictable.

During the never-ending treks between my parents' homes in Queens and the Bronx, and eventually Queens to New Jersey, I discovered the magic of "same songs". In the early years of these trips, I had to listen to whatever my parental units and I could agree upon. Separately, they both indulged me by letting us listen to my favorite of our shared albums pretty regularly. With Mom, it was always Carole King, and with Dad, Billy Joel. But when Sony dropped the Walkman on the world, what music meant to me would completely level up.

I loved my first Walkman. It was a basic black rectangle a little bigger than what I could wrap my hand around and the headphones were simple silver metal with back plastic ear bugs covered by very thin, orange foam. I would eventually upgrade that first Walkman right along with Sony to a yellow waterproof one which would still be by today's standards a bulky beast. Nonetheless, that first Walkman made those intolerantly long rides in traffic to and fro every weekend go from something that I dreaded to my favorite time of the week, because all of a sudden I had auditory autonomy. Having a Walkman meant a socially acceptable, dare I say even trendy, way to control my auditory input. With my headphones on and music playing, I could tune out the boring adult conversation in the front seat, the nonstop horns blaring, and the irritating tick-tick-tick of the turn signals and enjoy whatever music suited my needs that day. Gone was the compromise on listening material and, in addition, I could now listen to my favorite songs over and over and over again, without having to beg someone for permission. And it was on those car rides with my private musical library that I learned the regulating power of music.

Eventually, my Walkman became a Discman and again it was a huge upgrade. With the move to CDs, we got an amazing bonus, the loop button. This invention, clearly spawned by an unknown Autistic, was pure magic. Looping my favorite stim songs with one button and not having to inaccurately rewind a cassette was my absolute favorite part of the Discman upgrade years. The ability to loop those songs endlessly led me to discover the ultimate source of self-regulation, same songs. Like safe foods, same songs are favored songs that Autistics find satisfying. Sometimes it's the melody, sometimes it's the rhythm, and sometimes the lyrics, and sometimes all three that seem to hit me just right, and it is so regulating that I will return to these same songs on repeat as a regular source of calm. Same songs are still one of my preferred ways to stay regulated. And in addition to same songs, the portability of both devices meant I could access a method of regulation a lot more often and in many more locations, like while running errands, in the shower, and during school breaks.

For Autistics, self-regulatory activities often serve as a means of recharging, akin to how others might use sleep, something that notoriously evades neurodivergent folks. My experiences with my Walkman are a clear example. It was not just a device for listening to music to me, but a portable tool for emotional and sensory regulation—like an assistive aid. More recently, devices like cell phones and handheld video games have replaced the Walkman and Discman, yet to Autistics the core motivation for their use remains the same: self-regulation. Portable digital devices are more than just a distraction or entertainment to us; they are essential tools that help us manage sensory overload, emotional stress, and mental exhaustion, often providing a very necessary refuge in a world that can be extremely demanding.

Parents are commonly told to limit their child's screen time, but this discounts the way Autistic people use those screens. Limiting screen time or headphone time for Autistic individuals can disrupt crucial self-regulatory practices and lead to more frequent meltdowns, shutdowns, mutism, burnout, and worse. This restriction often forces us to adhere to external schedules for when we can regulate and teaches us to disregard our intrinsic needs for regulation. Such limitations not only disregard Autistic needs, but also teach us a harmful lesson: that others have the authority to dictate when and how our needs are met.

Limiting screen time can compound our regulatory challenges and unnecessarily increase our discomfort. Like masking, this adds to our overall burden, teaches us to ignore our own dys-regulation and discomfort, and ingrains in us dangerous people-pleasing behaviors. Autistic kids are three to four times more likely than non-Autistic kids to experience sexual victimization (Trundle et al., 2023). This increased risk is due, in part, to the fact we teach Autistic kids to ignore their own comfort for the benefit of the neuromajority. We are told implicitly and repeatedly that the space is not for us and in order to participate we have to ignore our instincts. It's no surprise then that sexual abusers see us as better targets for their grooming.

Understanding and respecting the importance of self-regulatory activities, including unrestricted access to devices, is crucial in supporting the well-being and autonomy of Autistic individuals.

Regulation can also come from lowering anxiety levels. As I got older, I had a huge amount of anxiety surrounding socializing with my peers. I mostly had mastered adult interactions, but as peer socialization became more complex, I felt more and more like an outsider. My desire to fit in socially spurred my special interest in television and movies. I loved watching the actors' facial expressions and body movements and I was fascinated with their ability to understand each other's feelings and responses. How did these actors learn to play the role of human beings? How did they decide which gestures to use and when to make eye contact? It was the need for these practiced social skills that drove me to want to be an actor.

From 8 years old to 18, I would dedicate my extracurricular time to learning to play human through endless hours of acting classes. I didn't know that's what I was doing, but as we dug into exercises that required practicing facial expressions in the mirror and others that allowed only fake language and relied on the tone of voice to communicate information, I was getting more practice at the parts of social interactions that I didn't naturally rely upon. Plus, I found out quickly that the one place where my "odd" personality wasn't an issue was with my fellow weirdos in the theater world.

The ten years I spent focusing on acting were formidable ones. I needed those acting exercises outside of the theater as much as I did in it. And more than that, I had craved the sense of belonging that the theater community gave me since I was watching the Deaf kids use sign language with each other. I found my self-confidence in those theater classes, right along with the skill set to publicly speak that I use in my career today. As a theater kid, I tapped right into my ability to memorize information when learning new scripts, leaving me with plenty of time to perfect the walk, talk, and look of a new character, a skill I would also use to mask like an expert for many years as an undiagnosed Autistic. My theater friends were my support system, my safe place to experiment with my identity. The theater world was how I came to learn exactly what belonging feels like.

Motivated by the desire to alleviate anxiety, I found myself seeking social skills through acting. This was particularly effective for me, as Autistics usually acquire knowledge and skills best through hands-on experience. Social skills are no exception. We require ample practice for us to navigate the complexities of social interactions effectively. It's through this practical engagement that we discern our likes and dislikes in social settings. However, it's crucial to recognize the importance of not imposing a specific form of socializing on Autistic individuals. Social interaction has no definitive right or wrong approach, and the quantity or style of socializing should not be dictated by external expectations. Autistics inherently socialize differently, and this diversity in social interaction should be respected and understood, rather than forcing us to conform to mainstream norms.

The Autistic approach to socialization and communication often diverges from what is typically valued by the neuromajority. For instance, nonverbal cues such as body language, tone of voice, and eye contact are not prioritized in the way Autistic individuals communicate. Instead, we place a greater emphasis on the precise use of words, relying heavily on verbal communication to convey our thoughts and feelings, often relying more heavily on the written word than speech. While we can learn and mimic nonverbal communication techniques, they do not come naturally to us, and the significance placed on them is often something we simply cannot understand. Similarly, our preferences in relationships and social interactions often differ from the neuromajority. Autistic friendships may require less frequent interaction to remain strong, and we often find that we need smaller, less frequent social engagements as compared to non-Autistics. Our unique approach to socializing and building relationships may be different, but it is by no means less than or deficient. It is simply the unrecognized reflection of the diverse variety of human social needs and interactions.

I cannot emphasize enough how important finding self-regulation methods without judgment is for Autistics. For us, it is not only how we regulate ourselves but also how we find Autistic joy. Often when we engage in activities that bring us genuine happiness we are met with societal misunderstandings and external pressures to do our joy differently. The ability to self-regulate, whether through specific hobbies, routines, or stimming behaviors, is vital to our maintaining emotional and psychological well-being. Similarly, the pursuit of Autistic joy, those moments of pure contentment and engagement in activities that resonate deeply with our Autistic sensibilities, is a fundamental aspect of living a thriving and fulfilling life. Autistics should be free from judgment and need to conform to neurotypical standards in this pursuit of regulation, balance, and potential joy. It is essential to recognize and embrace the diversity in how Autistic individuals experience and interact with the world. Celebrating these differences, rather than viewing them through a lens of deficiency or abnormality, fosters an environment of acceptance and understanding. Such an approach not only validates the experiences of Autistic individuals but also highlights the myriad ways in which joy and contentment can be found and expressed.

For many of us, the pursuit of a happy and satisfying life can be a long journey, but if it's one informed by self-knowledge and freedom from judgment, we are capable of meeting our goals and creating a life we don't feel like we constantly need a vacation from. This I know from experience, and I'll share that and where I find my Autistic joy in our next and final chapter together.

12
A life you don't need a vacation from

Growing up an undiagnosed Autistic in New York City certainly had its challenges. It was a loud life from which I was always seeking escape. During my pre-identification years, I didn't stand a chance at successful regulation. There was just too much that was out of my control, and I was missing all the clues to happiness that knowing I was Autistic would have given me. Instead of being taught to tweak my life according to my needs and make my environment work with me, my childhood experiences taught me to tweak myself instead, that I was the one that was broken, didn't fit, and needed to be someone else to be valued.

I didn't know it then, but the moment that autism entered my world was the beginning of a new life for me. In that instant, for the first time in over 30 years, I was able to see that not only was there potential for my life to be different, but that it could be a life I could enjoy, one that I wasn't constantly wishing for a break from.

It was about a year after that sunny day in May with my mom that I began work on building that possible life. It all started with an idea, a giant but hopeful goal for the future. Armed with the new self-knowledge my diagnosis provided, I set out on a new mission: to create a life that I didn't need a vacation from.

What I had come to realize in that first year was that so much of what I pressured myself to achieve didn't come from me at all. I was pushing myself to Autistic burnout time and again in endless attempts to attain other people's wishes, wants, and dreams for me, instead of my own. I was using all my precious energy and time to pursue a life that I didn't even really want and then continuously beating myself up inside for my inability to get there. It needed to stop, and I needed to redefine my life.

I began by thinking about the big trigger words in my life—the ones that carried the baggage of other people's expectations with them. Words like happiness, family, love, and my most dreaded word, success. What did it mean to me to be successful? What did it mean to have success? Was success truly the end goal of living, or was it happiness? When I broke down what that word meant to me, I realized that what I truly believed success to be was not the version of success that I was helplessly chasing and so epically failing to catch.

I had been in pursuit of an endless list of "things" that would prove my success to the outside world. Chasing degrees, jobs, relationships, anything that would show the world I was "successful", but no matter how many boxes I ticked, I was still consistently miserable. It was time for me to redefine success on my terms and put all of that energy and time I had been using to guess at life into pursuing this new self-defined version of success. It was time to find that inner voice I had silenced for so long and ask myself what success meant to me, and me alone.

It didn't take long to see that what success meant to me was very different from the version of success that had been spoon-fed to me by a world fueled by sameness. Success to me wouldn't look like the "right" job, house, or husband, but instead, success to me would be to feel like I fit in my life instead of shoving myself into a life that I didn't even like. Success for me would be living a life aligned with my values and waking up most days happy about opening my eyes. To me, success could not be quantified, tallied, or compared using things, but was instead a subjective journey that we are all on to reach a personal goal or to fulfill a purpose. Success is not one thing to many people, but rather many things to many people. And with that understanding of myself, life suddenly went from being a competition with others for things to being a uniquely individual aspirational journey of self-discovery. It was so obvious. How had I missed it for so many years?

Of course, my success would never look like other people's success, and it was time to stop wanting it to. And with that, it was time to chase the life that I wanted for myself: a life that I was happy to wake up in, a life that met MY expectations of a self-defined, successful life, a life I didn't need a vacation from.

The first year after identification I spent looking back on my life and wondering about all the relationships, jobs, and other experiences that I could have done differently if I had known I was Autistic sooner. I wondered how many of my bad choices, poor decisions, mistakes, and traumas were the result of being uninformed about my neurology. Like most of us who are diagnosed late in life, I spent that year cycling through my life and revisiting every one of those memories through the lens of autism, deciding about each one whether I was at fault or was it related to being Autistic. Needless to say, I spent that year full of rage and even more sadness. I yelled and cried for little me, who had muddled through the world for over three decades feeling lost, alone, and broken, and as I processed, I realized just how unkind I had always been to myself. How for years, whether or not it was true, I blamed myself for every hardship I encountered, every failed relationship, and every job I left behind. It was always my fault for being odd, without a single consideration for any other possibility.

I had come to understand that in the first 36 years of my life, I was taught that my needs and wants were "wrong", and that my natural instincts must be suppressed in favor of the "right" behavior. Without any direct instruction, the world had taught me that anything coming from my authentic self was not to be trusted. And the worst part? I believed every bit of it.

Today, I can tell you that none of that was true, except for how unkind I had been to myself, and that since then I have carefully, slowly, and with intention, deconstructed my life, and rebuilt it with all my new self-knowledge as my guide. I have methodically stripped away as many of the challenges imposed by societal expectations as possible, knowing they were built on the "shoulds" of others. And I have successfully rebuilt myself a life layered in all that I know about myself because of autism and let that guide me to my goals. I have spent hours upon hours reading personal development books, listening to podcasts, and watching TED talks on quality of life and how to achieve it. But I kept running into the same problem with all of it. No matter where I looked for personal development that suited me, none of it seemed to work for me because it was all by the neuromajority, for the neuromajority, and Autistics are guided by different motivating factors. But I knew I was onto something as some bits and pieces from each source sort of made sense, despite no single source being a great fit.

And that's when I had what I call an Autistic epiphany.

All of a sudden, I was able to see the pattern in all of the books, and that a lot of the things discussed were repeated no matter the source. It was all there; it just wasn't in a format that worked for my experiences or my brain. So, I went back through everything I had researched, ditched what wasn't working, and fine-tuned what was. Then, each day I took one small step forward to creating the life of my dreams. And I am thrilled to share that after almost a decade of dedication, I did it. I created a life so opposite of where I started from that it is wholly unrecognizable, and so am I.

Gone from life are the long work hours and night shifts to avoid rush hour in New York City. Gone are the noisy highways and lines for EVERYTHING. Gone is the bleakness of winter and the humidity of summer. Gone, too, is the angry and sad woman who suffered through 36 years on this planet.

Gone is the miserable lump of a human who communicated solely in sarcasm. Gone is the desire to be gone. In her place lives the real me, my authentic self. The one I spent so much energy masking to survive now lives freely and openly in a life that the old me wouldn't even dare to dream of.

The years of pain and struggle I went through could have been so different if my parents had access to and could have embraced the information in this book. This is not a complaint. I know they did the best with the information they had and, considering the era, I probably could not have had a more accommodating mom, but we DO know more now, and you can do better for your kid, so they don't end up a burned-out teenager on a 20-year quest to come back to themselves.

Each day that I wake up in this life, I am grateful. Grateful to still be here, grateful to be Autistic, and, most of all, grateful to be me. Grateful that every single moment of the blood, sweat, and tears it took to get here was worth it, but I want Autistic kids and their parents to know it doesn't have to be this way.

It was a lot of work to rebuild my life and my identity. And though I wouldn't change much about my journey, there are a few things that would have made it all just a bit easier.

To begin with, though being sensory sensitive can often be painful and overwhelming, it can also come with a unique set of advantages. Autistics like me with heightened sensory awareness tend to experience the world in a deeply enriched way, which allows us to notice subtleties that others usually miss. This can lead to a greater appreciation of art, music, and nature, as we can perceive nuances in color, texture, sound, and flavor that are less apparent to others. Sensory-sensitive people also often exhibit heightened emotional empathy, as our keen perception enables us to pick up on smaller emotional cues. This makes many of us excellent listeners, as well as compassionate friends and partners. Moreover, our sensitivities can foster creativity and innovation, as we have rich sensory experiences to draw from for inspiration. So, while sensory sensitivity definitely has its challenges, it also opens the door to a world rich in detail and depth of experience and can even be a regular source of Autistic joy.

Like all human beings, it is essential to our well-being for Autistics to experience our version of joy. For us, that may come from mastering a new language or creating a brilliant bit of code. It might be the result of freely stimming to your favorite same song or hyper-focusing on a newly discovered special interest. Regardless of how "odd" the source may seem to the outside world, Autistic individuals deserve to experience joy in its purest form as much as the next human. Moreover, our brains and bodies NEED joy to regulate and function at our best. That's right, WE NEED AUTISTIC JOY.

Fortunately for all of us, Autistic joy is best experienced when shared with others, as mutually joyful activities have exponential potential to offset a lot of dysregulation. Joy contributes to not only our overall well-being but also our ongoing satisfaction with our lives and relationships. Joy, a positive emotion, when experienced, not only uplifts our spirits but also has profound benefits for our mental and physical health, and when this joy is shared, its benefits magnify. Shared joy creates strong bonds between individuals while fostering a sense of belonging and mutual regulation that is fundamental to human relationships. It acts as a social glue, bringing people together in a way that transcends any differences. In moments of shared joy, whether in celebrations, communal achievements, or simple everyday inter-actions, we find a powerful antidote to feelings of isolation and dysregulation.

Creating opportunities for Autistic joy isn't difficult and we truly appreciate it when others initiate joyful activities on our behalf. Below are a few ways that you can encourage Autistic joy as a regulation tool.

Look for big challenges

Nothing creates joy like a deep dive into an Autistic special inter-est. We get set up for that joyful feeling of accomplishment by taking on a new project, skill, or hobby that calls to us. It helps if it's something we have wanted to do for a long time. Encourage your kid to challenge themselves to do things like completing a collection, or logging a full data set, or finishing reading a set of encyclopedias like I did. We find joy in collecting and comple-tion in our special interests, so help us set a challenge and track our progress. When we are engaged in our special interests, we find joy.

Actively seek inspiration

As we talked about in the book, Autistics have hyper-connected brains that process more information. This means our sensitivi-ties are more triggering, but also more glimmering! Autistic joy comes from pleasurable sensory experiences in equal propor-tion to our misery coming from miserable sensory experiences. Seek out activities that are known to elicit joy for Autistics, like going out into nature or listening to music. Actively pursue that which stretches perception and challenges perspective and keep a log of what did and didn't spark a glimmer. When we are most inspired, we find joy.

Make space for play

Does your kid love jumping in puddles in a thunderstorm or getting dirty in the garden? Maybe they like to lick the spoon clean while baking. It's easy as a parent to want to set limits and say no. No, you can't come into the house with muddy boots. No, you can't put your germy hands in our chocolate chip cookies! But I encourage you to look for the lessons. It's easy to forget the importance of play. Create the time and space in your family life to dig out those dress-up clothes and board games, be silly, and play. When we play freely, we find joy.

Encourage your child's instincts

When we take the time to focus on our own needs and follow our instincts, joy comes more easily. Set up time to get away from the "noise of life" and do something just for fun. As an adult, you know this, but as an Autistic receiving messages all day that our instincts are wrong, it is hard to trust ourselves. As a parent, it's your job to foster that trust. Help your kid find the stuff that recharges them and leaves them open to experience happiness. Teach your child the practice of making it a priority to listen to themselves. When we trust ourselves, we find joy.

Rebuilding my life Autistically with regulation and joy as priorities meant for me that I needed to get out of New York as soon as possible. As a sensory-sensitive Autistic, New York and I will never be a good fit. Living there for decades taught me an irreplaceable resilience that I hope to never need to rely on again.

It is a loud city with too many people for me and not enough open quiet space with views of the sky. I left New York first for the Rocky Mountains of Colorado for a few years and then settled at the base of the Highlands of Maine, just outside of Bangor, in the heart of Stephen King territory. With family and friends still in New York, I occasionally return for visits and work trips. I meet each trip there with apprehension and leave feeling grateful I now know how to take care of myself so much better.

I have activities that bring me Autistic joy built into my routine and am surrounded by more pets than most people can manage. Six cats, four dogs, two snakes, and a tortoise, along with my husband, make up my pack. We are a happy and regulated crew that prioritizes couch snuggles and outside adventures, but also each other's needs. My home is mostly quiet, really boring, and exactly the way I had always wished life could be.

As I close this final chapter, I reflect on my journey not just as an individual who navigated life undiagnosed but with the hope that I can make the journey easier for families like yours. Of course, your journey is unique, filled with its own set of challenges and joys, but maybe some of the lessons from my life can offer you insights into a world that might sometimes seem puzzling.

When I told my mom that I was Autistic, she told me she wished she had known. She wanted to know what she could have done better. I know my mom did her best, and if you are reading this book, it's clear you are too. It's important you know that. Your child, much like I was, might be seeking their own path in a world that feels overwhelmingly loud and chaotic. It's crucial to recognize that their way of experiencing life is deeply valid and meaningful. As a parent, your role is to guide them, to help them understand themselves, and to create an environment where they can thrive.

Teach your child to embrace their autism as a part of who they are, not something that needs to be fixed or hidden. Encourage them to pursue what brings them joy and comfort, whether it's a deep dive into their favorite subjects, sensory play, or quiet time with a beloved book or toy. Celebrate their successes, no matter how small they may seem, and understand that their definition of success might look different from yours—and that's okay.

Create a safe space for them to express their feelings and frustrations. Understand that their struggles and meltdowns are not acts of defiance but expressions of being overwhelmed in a world not designed for their unique wiring. Equip them with tools and strategies to cope with sensory overload and social challenges.

Most importantly, do the thing my mom absolutely got right: let your child know they are loved and accepted for who they are. Your acceptance and understanding are the greatest gifts you can give them. It will empower them to grow into their authentic selves, unburdened by the need to conform to a world that doesn't always understand them.

Remember, your journey with your Autistic child is a shared one. It's about learning, growing, and adapting together. It's about finding joy in the little things and celebrating the world through their unique lens. You will get a lot wrong along the way, and so will your child, but your support and love will be the guiding light in their journey, helping them navigate life's challenges and embrace their true selves so they build a life they don't need a vacation from.

It is with a message that resonates with both urgency and hope: I want to leave you, the reader, deeply infused with a motivation to learn all that you can about the Autistics in your life. Autistic individuals are not delicate creatures to be observed from a distance; we are vibrant, complex humans with a rich tapestry of experiences, thoughts, and emotions that may be different from yours, but are no less valuable. There is an immeasurable depth and diversity to be found in the Autistic experience that often goes unrecognized and misunderstood. We, as Autistics, have so much we could share with the world, so many stories, perspectives, and insights that could profoundly enrich the lives of all of those around us. But we can only share when we are allowed to be unapologetically ourselves, without the constraints of societal norms and the assumptions and judgment that come with it.

But that's enough reading about all of this, it's time to get out there and put some of it into practice. Seriously...stop reading and go create some Autistic joy in your family!

Suggested discussion topics

Here are some questions to facilitate thoughtful conversation and deeper understanding of the book's insights:

1. Exploring sensory sensitivities: How does Hector's emphasis on sensory sensitivities contribute to our understanding of the daily experiences of Autistic individuals? Discuss the importance of recognizing and accommodating these sensitivities in both personal and public spaces.

2. Social invalidation and autism: Hector shares experiences of social invalidation due to her autism. How do these experiences highlight the challenges Autistic individuals face in social interactions and broader societal acceptance? Discuss strategies that can be employed to foster a more inclusive and understanding society.

3. Parental guidance and support: The book offers guidance to non-Autistic parents raising Autistic children. What are some key takeaways for parents in understanding and supporting their Autistic children's needs? Discuss the balance between advocating for one's child and empowering them to advocate for themselves.

References

Auel, J. M. (2002). *The Clan of the Cave Bear: Earth's Children, Book One* (Vol. 1). London: Bantam.

Baron-Cohen, S., Leslie, A. M., and Frith, U. (1985). Does the Autistic Child Have a 'Theory of Mind'? *Cognition*, 21(1), pp. 37–46.

Garfinkel, S. N., Seth, A. K., Barrett, A. B., Suzuki, K., and Critchley, H. D. (2016). Knowing Your Own Heart: Distinguishing Interoceptive Accuracy from Interoceptive Awareness. *Biological Psychology*, 104, pp. 65–74. Available at: https://pubmed.ncbi.nlm.nih.gov/25451381/ [Accessed 23 February 2024].

Grove, R., Hoekstra, R. A., Wierda, M., and Begeer, S. (2018). Special Interests and Subjective Wellbeing in Autistic Adults. *Autism Research: Official Journal of the International Society for Autism Research*, 11(5), pp. 766–775. Available at: https://doi.org/10.1002/aur.1931 [Accessed 23 February 2024].

Intriago, K. E. C., Rodríguez, L. M. A., and Cevallos, L. A. T. (2021). Specific Learning Difficulty: Autism, Dyscalculia, Dyslexia and Dysgraphia. *International Research Journal of Engineering, IT & Scientific Research*, 7(3), pp. 97–106. Available at: www.researchgate.net/publication/368002250_Specific_learning_difficulty_autism_dyscalculia_dyslexia_and_dysgraphia [Accessed 23 February 2024].

Kapp, S. K., Gillespie-Lynch, K., Sherman, L. E., and Hutman, T. (2013). Deficit, Difference, or Both? Autism and Neurodiversity. *Developmental Psychology*, 49(1), pp. 59–71.

Macdonald, D., Luk, G., and Quintin, E. M. (2022). Early Reading Comprehension Intervention for Preschoolers with Autism Spectrum Disorder and Hyperlexia. *Journal of Autism and Developmental Disorders*, 52, pp. 1652–1672. Available at: https://doi.org/10.1007/s10803-021-05057-x [Accessed 23 February 2024].

Miller, D., Rees, J., and Pearson, A. (2021). "Masking Is Life": Experiences of Masking in Autistic and Nonautistic Adults. *Autism in Adulthood: Challenges and Management*, 3(4), pp. 330–338. Available at: https://doi.org/10.1089/aut.2020.0083 [Accessed 23 February 2024].

Milton, D. E. M. (2012). On the Ontological Status of Autism: The 'Double Empathy Problem'. *Disability & Society*, 27(6), pp. 883–887.

Parish-Morris, J., Liberman, M. Y., Cieri, C., Herrington, J. D., Yerys, B. E., Bateman, L., Donaher, J., Pandey, J., Schultz, R. T., and Chatterjee, A. (2017). Linguistic Camouflage in Girls with Autism Spectrum Disorder. *Molecular Autism*, 8(1), Article 48. Available at: https://doi.org/10.1186/s13229-017-0164-6 [Accessed 23 February 2024].

Pearson, A. and Rose, K. (2021). A Conceptual Analysis of Autistic Masking: Understanding the Narrative of Stigma and the Illusion of Choice. *Autism in Adulthood*, 3(1), pp. 52–60.

South, M., Costa, A. P., and McMorris, C. (2021). Death by Suicide Among People With Autism: Beyond Zebrafish. *JAMA Network Open*, 4(1), e2034018. Available at: https://doi.org/10.1001/aut.2021.0021 [Accessed 23 February 2024].

Trundle, G., Jones, K. A., Ropar, D., and Egan, V. (2023). Prevalence of Victimisation in Autistic Individuals: A Systematic Review and Meta-Analysis. *Trauma, Violence, & Abuse*, 24(4), 2282–2296. Available at: https://doi.org/10.1177/15248380221093689 [Accessed 23 February 2024].

Wharmby, P. (2022). *What I Want to Talk About*. London: Jessica Kingsley Publishers.

Wilson, A. C. (2023). Cognitive Profile in Autism and ADHD: A Meta-Analysis of Performance on the WAIS-IV and WISC-V. *Archives of Clinical Neuropsychology*, [online] 39(4), pp. 498–515. Available at: https://doi.org/10.1093/arclin/acad073 [Accessed 23 February 2024].

Recommended reading

Cook, B. (2018). *Spectrum Women: Walking to the Beat of Autism*. London: Jessica Kingsley Publishers.

Price, D. (2022). *Unmasking Autism: Discovering the New Faces of Neurodiversity*. New York, NY: Harmony Books.

Prizant, B. M. (2015). *Uniquely Human: A Different Way of Seeing Autism*. New York, NY: Simon & Schuster.

Silberman, S. (2015). *NeuroTribes: The Legacy of Autism and the Future of Neurodiversity*. New York, NY: Penguin Random House.

Walker, N. (2021). *Neuroqueer Heresies: Notes on the Neurodiversity Paradigm, Autistic Empowerment, and Postnormal Possibilities*. Fort Worth, TX: Autonomous Press.

Index

Abnormal psychology. 8

Adulting skills. 7

Adult-oriented event. 62

Advocacy work. 14

Alexithymia. 71

Anorexia. 55

Autism; diagnosis. 81, 84;
females. 75; hEDS. 82; high
functioning. 15; impacts
on physical health. 82;
profound. 15; spectrum. 15;
strengths and challenges. 27

Autistic brains. 33, 86

Autistic burnout;
causes. 84; recovery. 85;
skills and abilities. 84; social
expectations. 4; symptoms. 85

Autistic experiences. 6, 16, 40, 62,
82, 108

Autistic females. 74

Autistic Info Dump. 13

Autistic joy. 96, 104

Autistic kids. 10, 93, 102

Autistic naivety. 41

Autistic traits. 74

Autistics; challenges. 104;
encourage child instincts.
105, 106; knowledge
and skills. 94; motivating
factors. 101; motivations
and preferences. 89; seek
inspiration. 104; sense
stimuli. 16; space for play. 105;
SPINS. 10; unexpected
changes. 48; version of
joy. 103

Avoidant/restrictive food intake
disorder (ARFID). 55

Blocking out sounds. 88

Chronic pain. 17

Clumsiness. 17

Data collection. 16

Deaf kids. 87, 94

Decision-making abilities. 71

Disabilities. 19, 20

Double empathy problem. 39

Dyscalculia. 19, 26

Dysregulation. 72

Ehlers-Danlos Syndrome
(hEDS). 82

Emotional experience. 71

Empowerment. 21, 50, 64, 107

Errands. 31–34

Exhaustion. 17

Explicit explanations. 40

Eye contact. 73

Firsthand experiences. 40

Gifted and talented
    programs. 19, 20

Hidden immunity. 70

High functioning autism. 15

Historical fiction. 23

Hyperfocus mode. 10

Hyperlexia. 2, 27

Hyperverbal hyperlexic. 3

Identity. 65, 77, 94, 102

Information Seeker. 13

Intense hobby. 10

Interoception. 71

Joyful activities. 103

Learning disability. 26

Life experiences. 40

Linear functioning. 21

Logical reasoning. 12

Magnetic resonance imaging
    (MRI). 79, 81

Masking. 17, 66, 74

Mental health; implications. 75;
    issues. 16

Migraines. 81, 86

Motormouth. 17

Mutism. 17

Negative language. 11

Negative sensory input. 65

Neurodiversity. 20

Neuromajority. 35, 73, 89, 95, 101

Neuro-normative social
    behavior. 74

Neurotypicals. 31

New York City Public Library
    system. 24

Non-autistic communication. 36

Non-autistics feel. 10

Nonverbal communication
    techniques. 95

NYC Public School system. 26

Obsessions. 11

Parental guidance. 44, 90

Pattern recognition. 16

Personal comfort. 66

Personal identity. 75

Physical discomfort. 85

Positive reinforcement. 16

Profound autism. 15

Quality of life. 10, 18, 101

Questioning authority. 35

Routines. 45

Safe foods. 53, 55, 57

Same songs. 91

Self-advocacy. 18

Self-awareness. 71

Self-esteem. 10, 75, 77

Self-regulation. 26, 72, 92

Sense of security. 49

Sensory experiences. 58

Sensory explosion. 61

Sensory overload. 16, 17, 66, 81,
    84, 85, 86, 92, 107

Sensory sensitivities. 63, 81, 86,
    102, 103

Sensory suppression. 17

Sign language. 88

Situational mutism. 16, 17

Smart kid. 20, 38

Social camouflaging. 74

Social communication. 17

Social interaction. 95

Social invalidation. 79

Social skills. 94

Societal expectations. 64

Special interests/SPINS. 9, 10, 11

Special needs kids. 87

Spectrum metaphor. 18

Spiky profile. 27

Static functioning. 21

Suicidal ideations. 1, 17

Temporary immunity. 70

Theory of Mind. 39

Troubled kids. 4, 38

Unhappiness. 17

Version of joy. 103

Version of success. 99

Wasted Food. 54

www.ingramcontent.com/pod-product-compliance
Lightning Source LLC
Chambersburg PA
CBHW061258220326
41599CB00028B/5696